T0129149

The Wonder of Life

A Series of Health Education Colouring Books

The Wonder of Life
A Series of Health Education Colouring Books

DAVID SACHS, MD

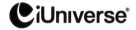

THE WONDER OF LIFE A SERIES OF HEALTH EDUCATION COLOURING BOOKS

iUniverse books may be ordered through booksellers or by contacting:

iUniverse
1663 Liberty Drive
Bloomington, IN 47403
www.iuniverse.com
1-800-Authors (1-800-288-4677)

Because of the dynamic nature of the Internet, any web addresses or links contained in this book may have changed since publication and may no longer be valid. The views expressed in this work are solely those of the author and do not necessarily reflect the views of the publisher, and the publisher hereby disclaims any responsibility for them.

Any people depicted in stock imagery provided by Thinkstock are models, and such images are being used for illustrative purposes only. Certain stock imagery © Thinkstock.

ISBN: 978-1-5320-3024-6 (sc)
ISBN: 978-1-5320-3025-3 (e)

Print information available on the last page.

iUniverse rev. date: 11/15/2017

YOUR ANATOMY

The purpose of the Wonder of Life series of health education colouring books about the human body and how it works is to provide children of all ages with the basics of health knowledge and to develop in them the natural sense of self-respect that awaits its rightful colourful expressions. With these books, children establish awareness of the kaleidoscopic energy in the magnificent patterns and designs that make up their precious human body.

It does not matter what colours the children use: what is important is that they give themselves the conscious attention that healthy bodily parts need to reinforce pride and respect while having a positive healthful effect on the whole body. Parents and teachers have the responsibility to give children every opportunity to experience daily exposure to each page of this fundamental series.

On every occasion have children actually visualize the exact location, form and function of the specific organ for the day's learning. While you allow them to freely colour their own expression of this, read aloud the simple text which accompanies each page, emphasizing whatever pleases you at the time. Through the sharing of this energy between a child and an adult, the entertaining appeal of colouring makes learning about the human body meaningful and fun.

When this series is used as part of children's everyday activities, you will be rewarded in knowing that they are receiving the foundation for a healthy life, and this will enable every other habit to be truly effective.

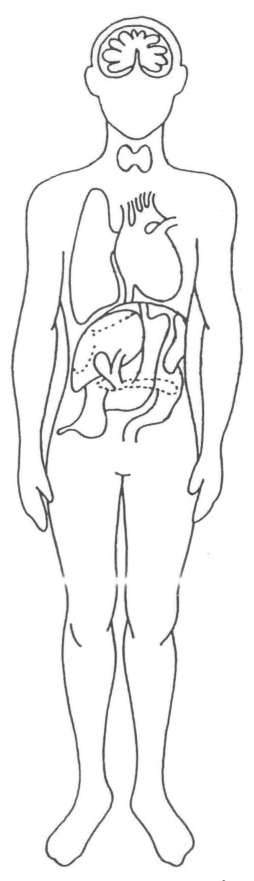

I am some of the parts
That make up your
Beautiful body

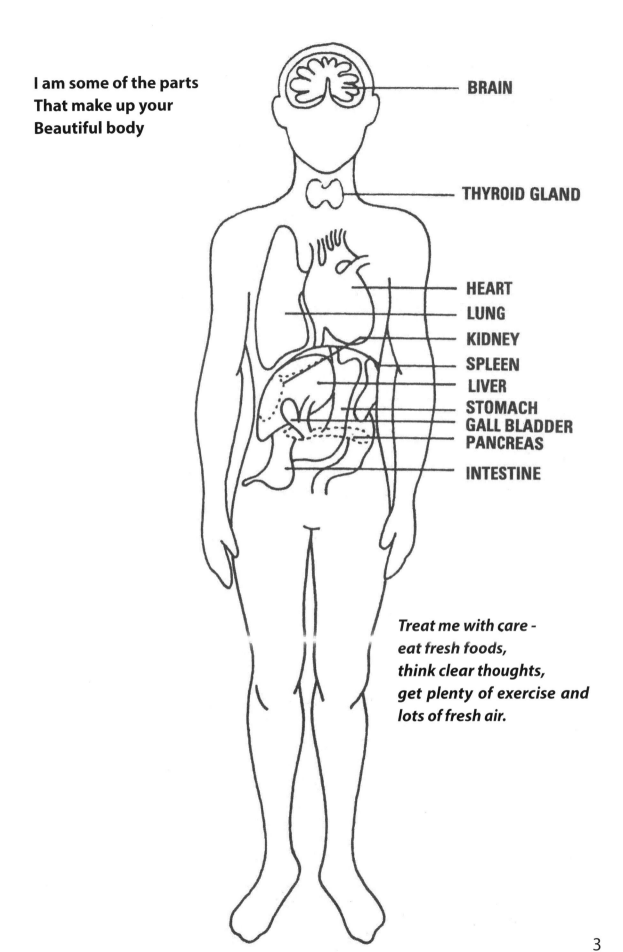

BRAIN

THYROID GLAND

HEART
LUNG
KIDNEY
SPLEEN
LIVER
STOMACH
GALL BLADDER
PANCREAS

INTESTINE

*Treat me with care -
eat fresh foods,
think clear thoughts,
get plenty of exercise and
lots of fresh air.*

3

HEART

OUTSIDE

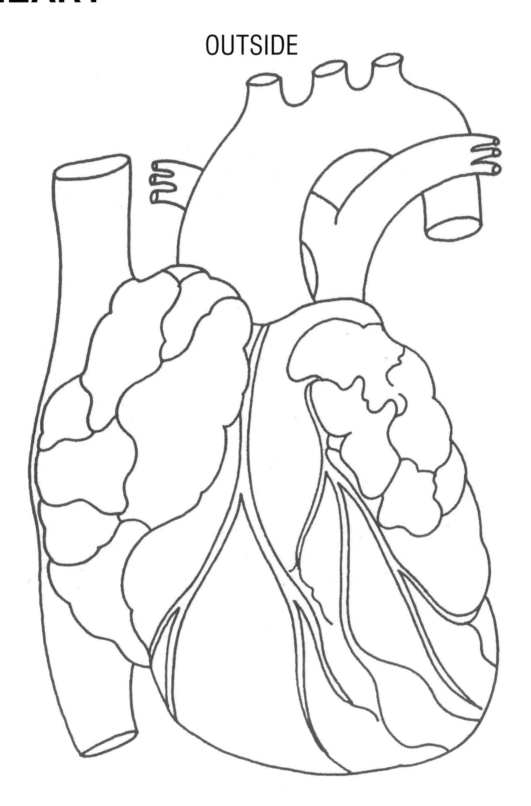

The heart is a muscle that pumps your blood

INSIDE

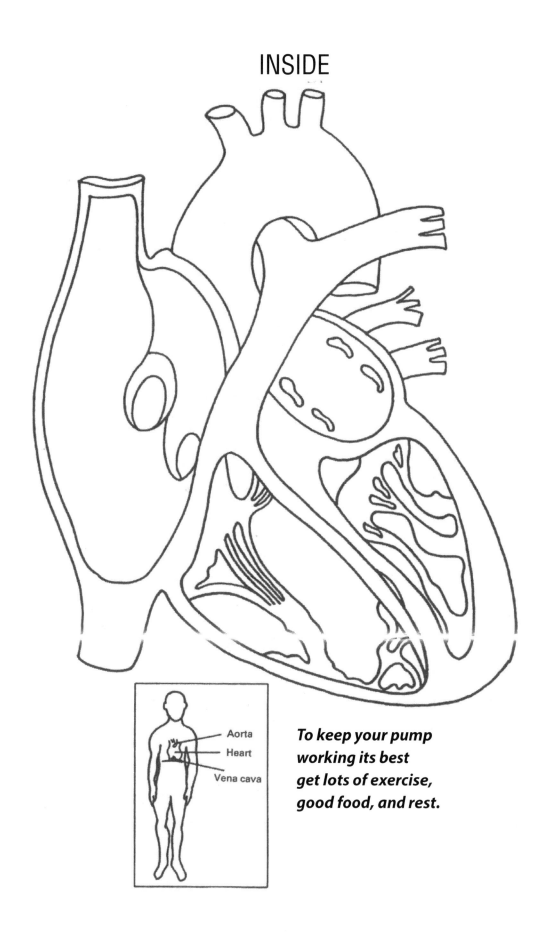

Aorta

Heart

Vena cava

To keep your pump working its best get lots of exercise, good food, and rest.

LUNG

OUTSIDE

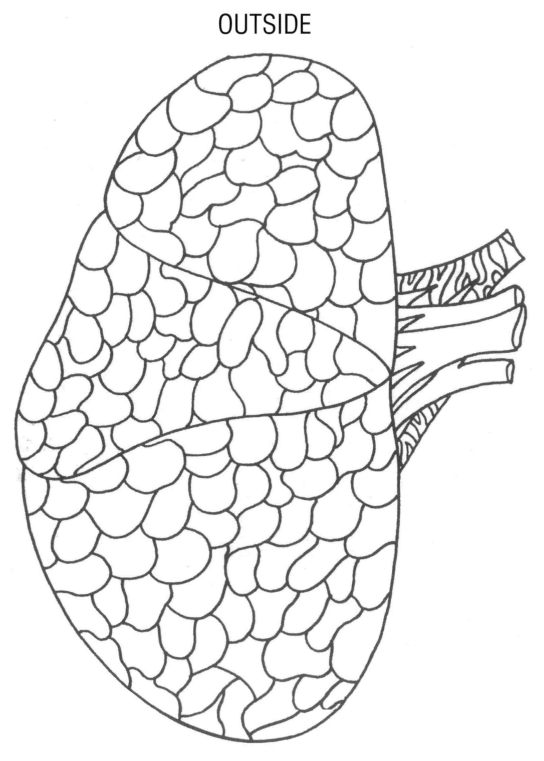

**The lung is a sac
where air enters
and leaves your body**

INSIDE

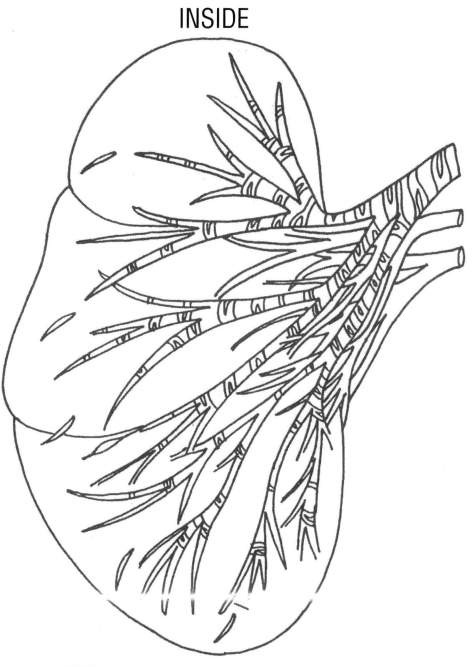

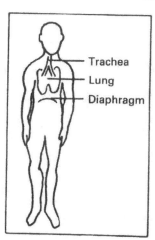

Trachea

Lung

Diaphragm

*Deep breathing
and pure air
will make your life
easier to bear.*

KIDNEY

OUTSIDE

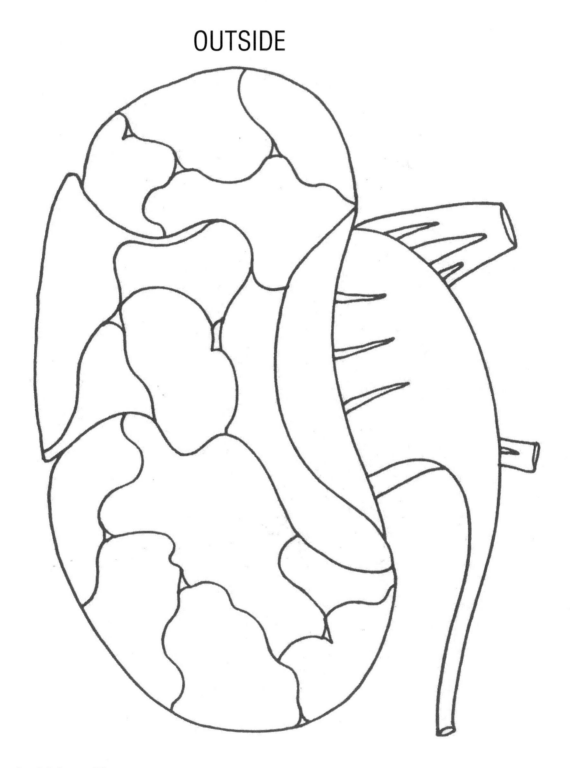

**The kidney filters
and cleans your blood
as it makes urine.**

INSIDE

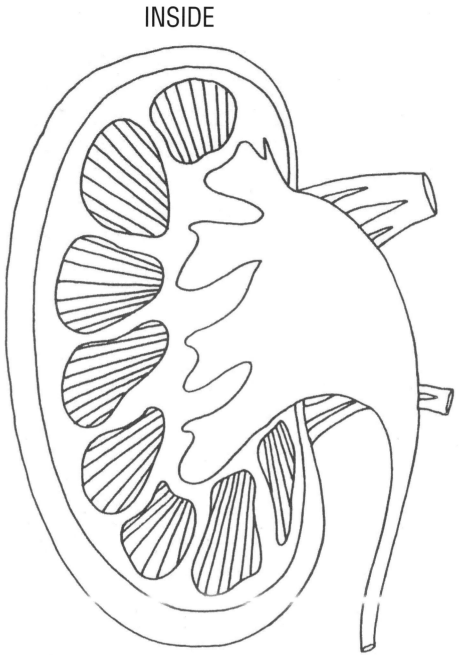

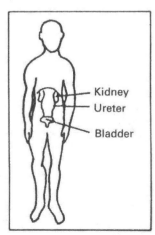

Kidney
Ureter

Bladder

*For kidneys calm and
waterworks fine
pure water you need
all of the time.*

BRAIN

OUTSIDE

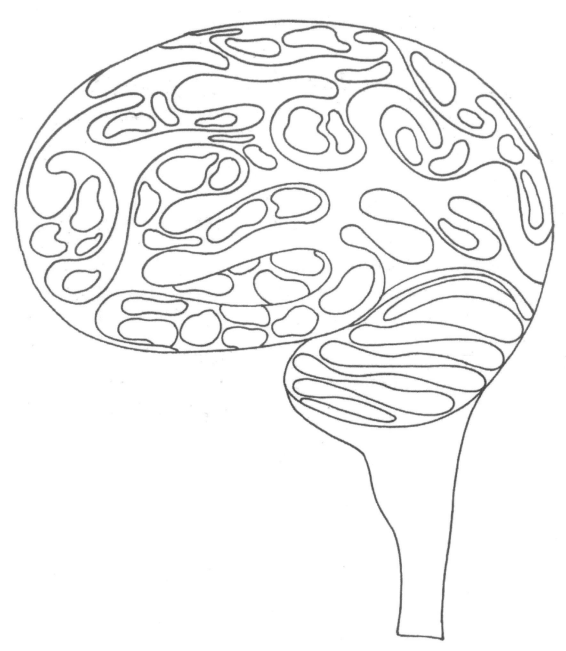

**The brain is your
living computer centre.**

INSIDE

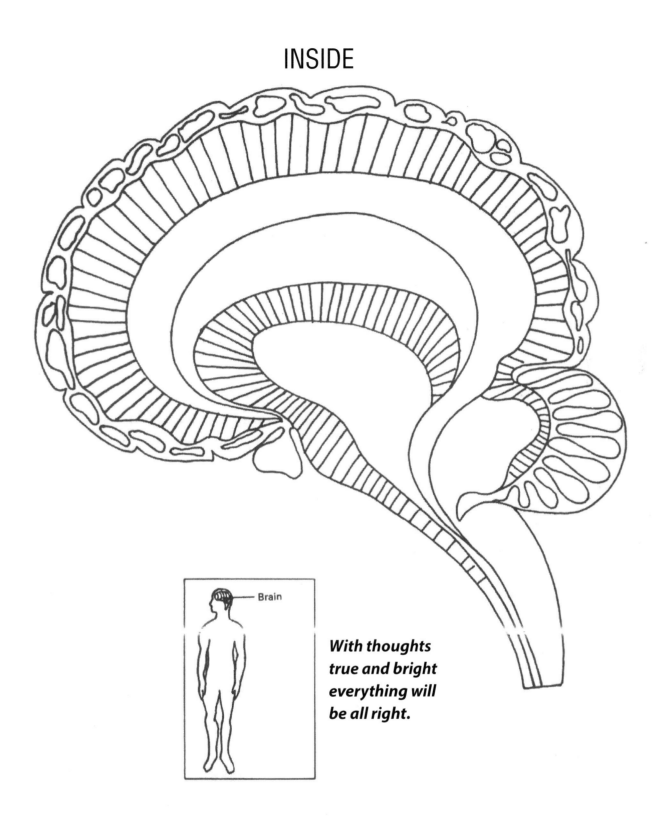

Brain

With thoughts true and bright everything will be all right.

STOMACH

OUTSIDE

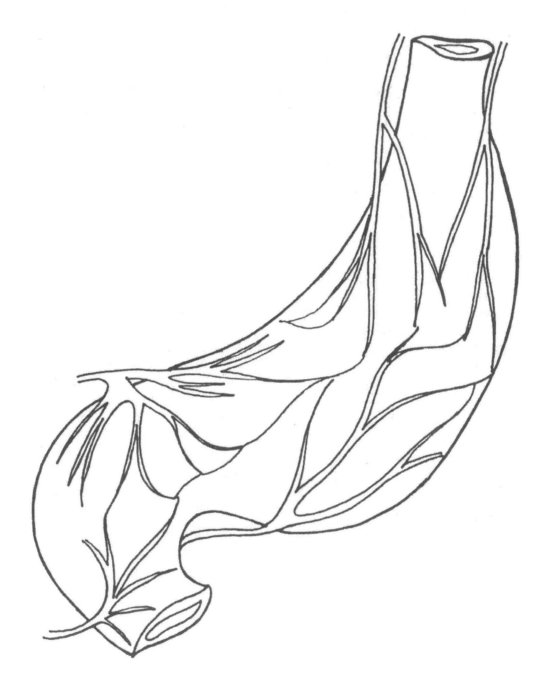

The stomach catches
the food you swallow
And prepares it for its
Journey.

INSIDE

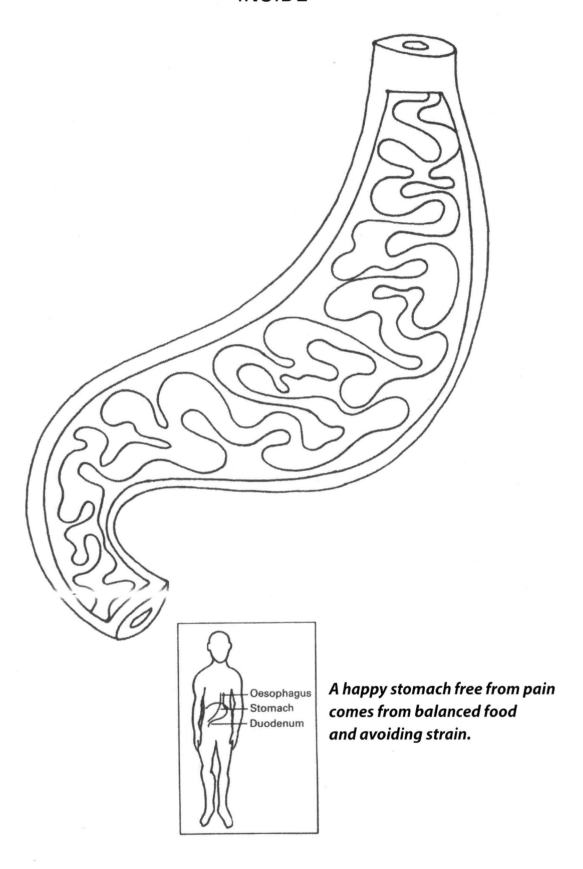

Oesophagus
Stomach
Duodenum

A happy stomach free from pain comes from balanced food and avoiding strain.

SPLEEN

The spleen exchanges
old blood for
new blood.

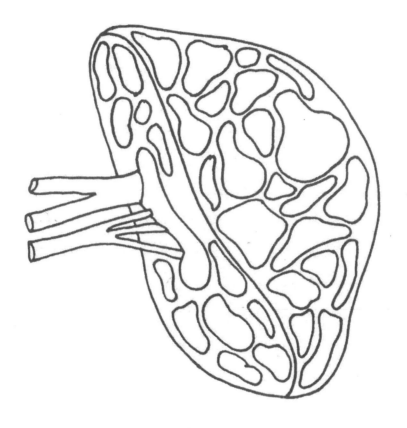

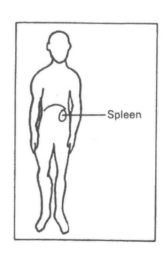

Spleen

*Eating fresh greens
with lots of iron
will keep the spleen from
blowing its siren.*

PANCREAS

The pancreas makes
chemicals that help
give your body energy.

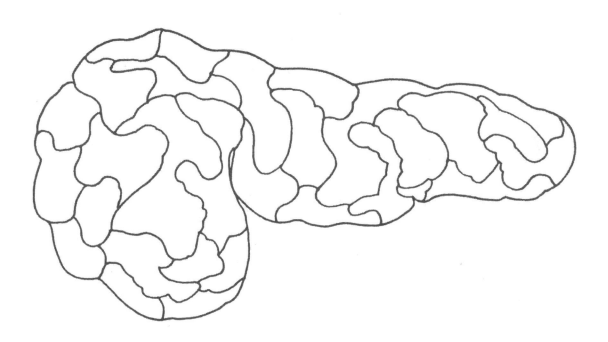

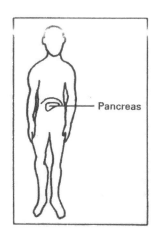

Pancreas

For enzymes gentle
and energy plus
give thanks every day
to your pancreas.

LIVER & GALL BLADDER

Your liver does many jobs to keep your body running smoothly.

Its neighbour the gall bladder stores its bile.

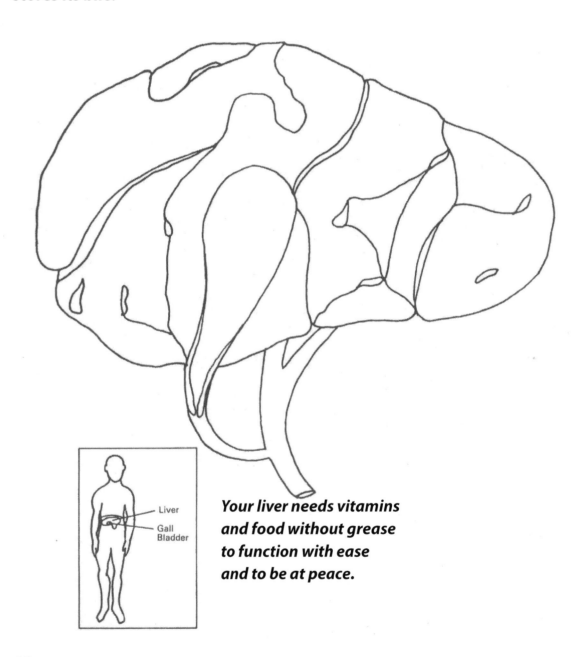

Liver

Gall
Bladder

Your liver needs vitamins and food without grease to function with ease and to be at peace.

INTESTINE

**The intestine carries
the food you eat
through your body.**

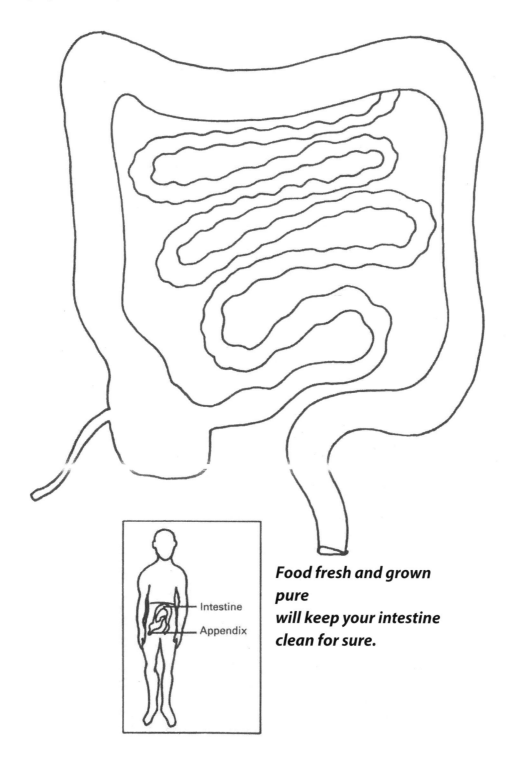

Intestine

Appendix

*Food fresh and grown
pure
will keep your intestine
clean for sure.*

THYROID GLAND

The thyroid gland makes a chemical that helps the body use the food' you eat.

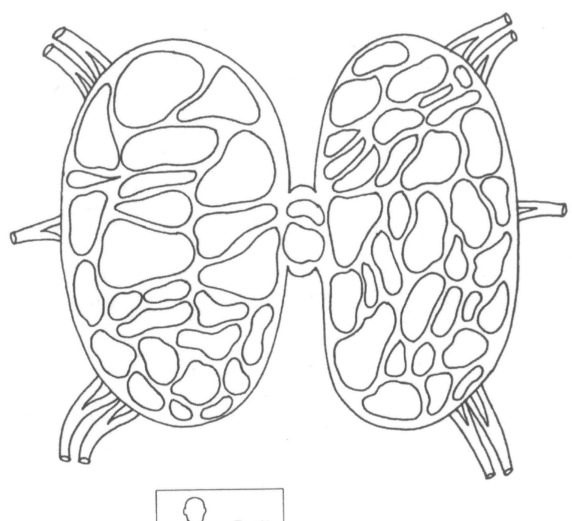

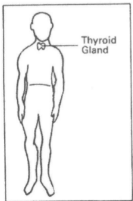

Thyroid Gland

Vigour comes from nutritious foods that keep your gland in its proper moods.

AORTA

The aorta is the main highway for blood in your body.

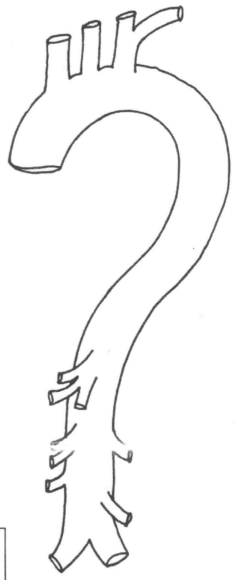

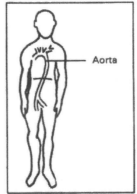

Aorta

Harmony exercise and rest will keep your bloods highway at its best.

EYE

OUTSIDE

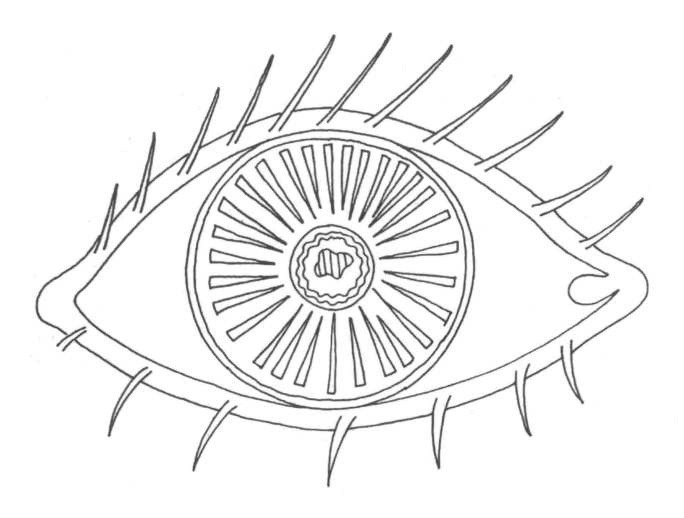

The eye is your camera, the way you see.

INSIDE (Side View)

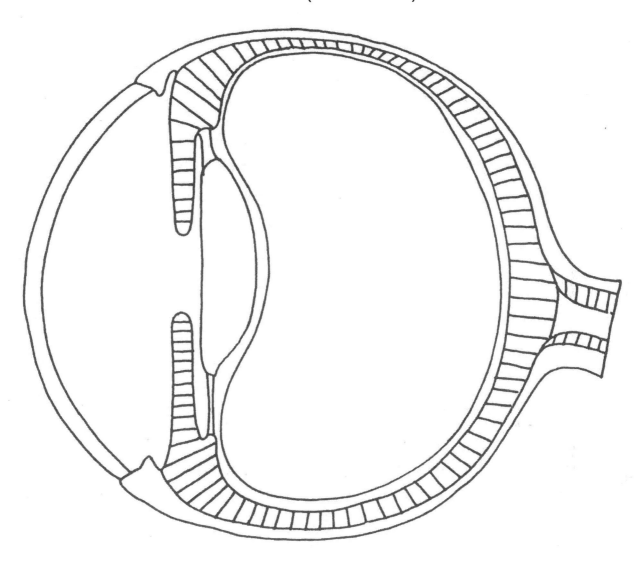

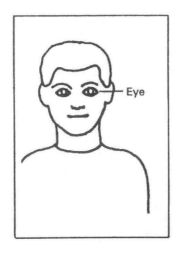

Eye

*If what you want
are eyes clear and bright
eat food like carrots
and read in good light.*

EAR

OUTSIDE

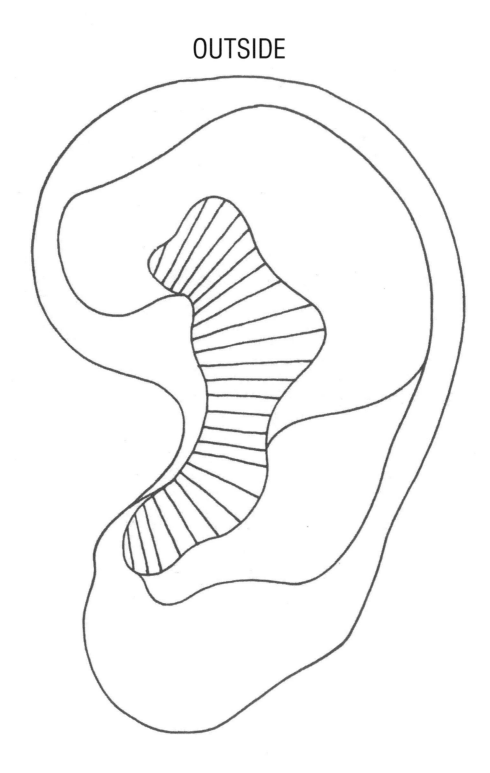

**The ear
picks up the sounds
you hear.**

INSIDE (Side View)

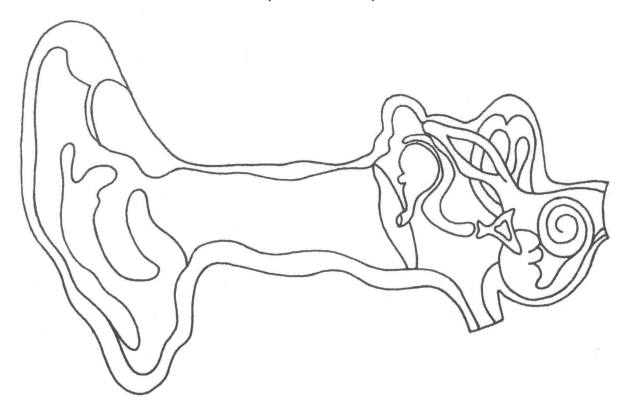

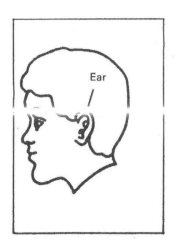

*Happy sounds will
be yours to hear
if dirt, toys and loud noises
are kept from your ear.*

NOSE

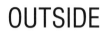
OUTSIDE

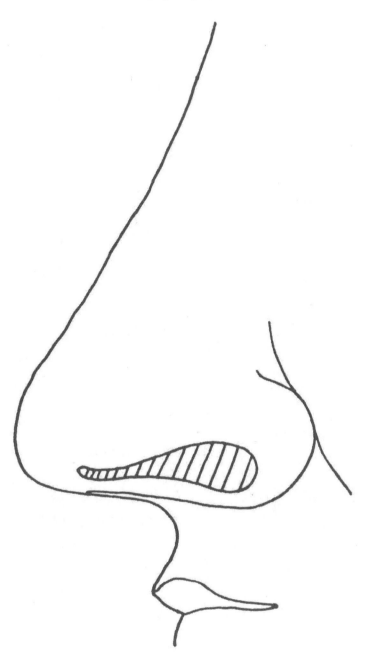

**The nose cleans
and warms the air
you breathe,
and lets you smell everything.**

24

INSIDE

—Nose

To keep your nose feeling right breathe clean air and avoid cold's bite.

BONE

**Your bones are
the building blocks
of your body.**

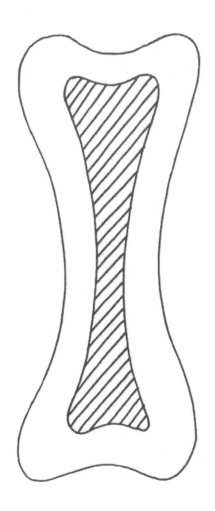

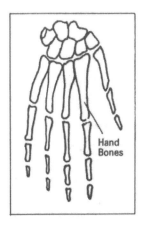

Hand
Bones

*Strong bones for your
delight
come with sunshine,
vitamin D and exercise
right.*

TOOTH

The tooth grinds food for your stomach to use.

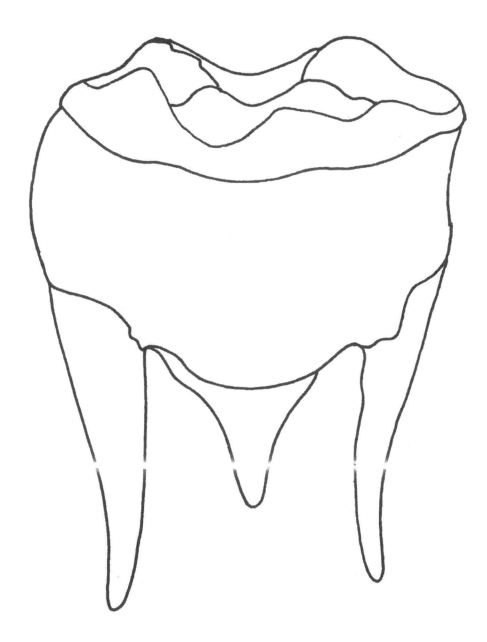

To keep your teeth free from decay, eat good foods and clean every day.

HAIR

**Your hair protects
your skin and
keeps you warm.**

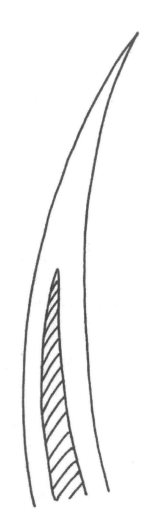

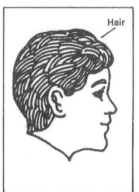

Hair

*The best way
to keep your hair
is to give it lots of care.*

28

NAIL

**You can use
your nails
to scratch an itch.**

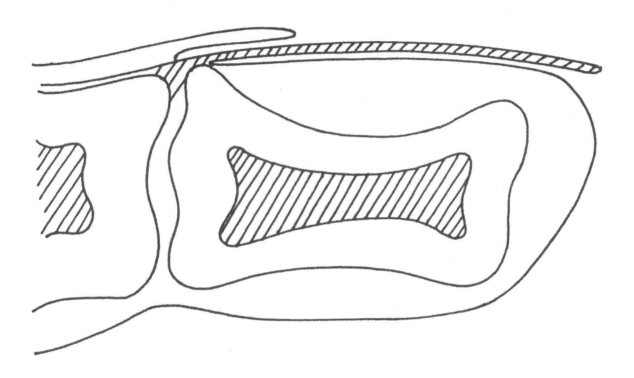

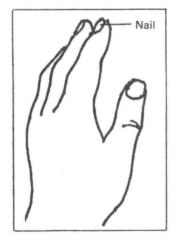

Nail

*Tender loving care is always fine-
for clean and natural nails that
shine.*

HOW OUR LIFE BEGINS
A CHILD'S INTRODUCTION TO THE HUMAN BODY

WONDER
OF LIFE

COLOURING BOOK

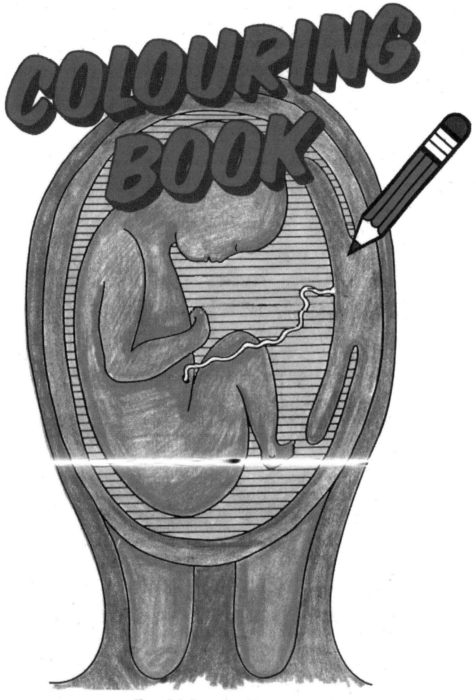

David Sachs M.D.

HOW OUR LIFE BEGINS

With these books, children establish awareness of the kaleidoscopic energy in the magnificent patterns and designs that make up their precious human body.

It does not matter what colours the children use: what is important is that they give themselves the conscious attention that healthy bodily parts need to reinforce pride and respect while having a positive healthful effect on the whole body.

Parents and teachers have the responsibility to give children every opportunity to experience daily exposure to each page of this fundamental series.

On every occasion have children actually visualize the exact location, form and function of the specific organ for the day's learning.

While you allow them to freely colour their own expression of this, read aloud the simple text which accompanies each page, emphasizing whatever pleases you at the time.

Through the sharing of this energy between a child and an adult, the entertaining appeal of colouring makes learning about the body meaningful and fun.

When this series is used as part of children's everyday activities, you will be rewarded in knowing that they are receiving the foundation for a healthy life, and this will enable every other health habit to be truly effective.

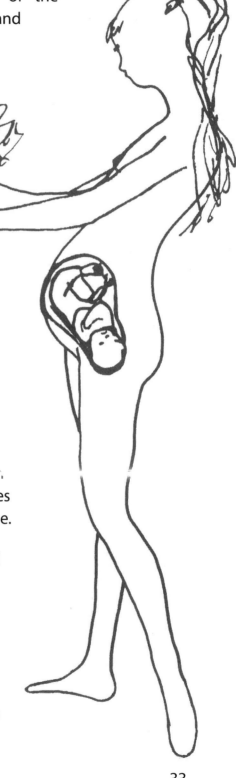

Little Anton could hardly wait to be born.

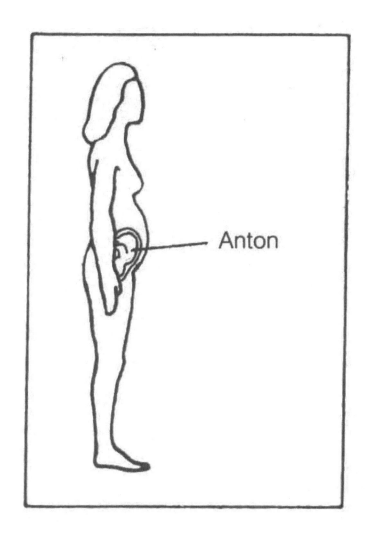

Anton

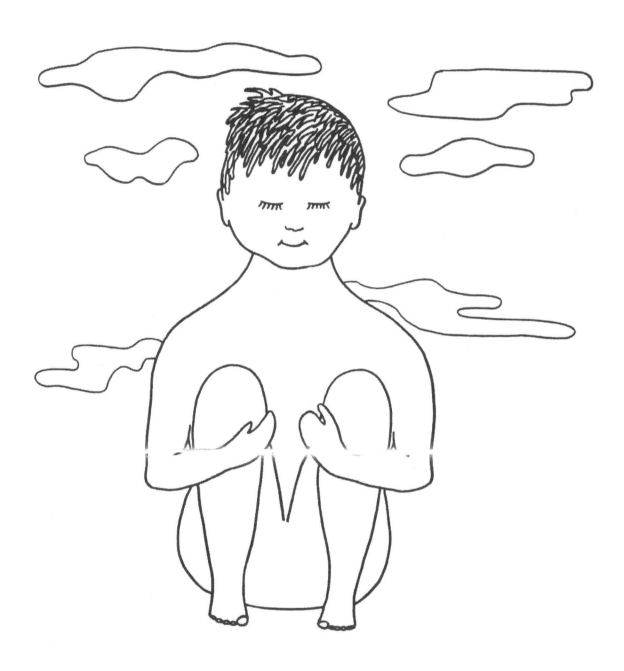

It was interesting for him to see what made man different from woman.

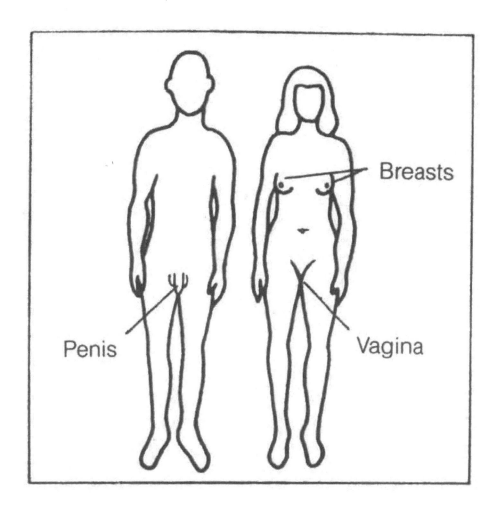

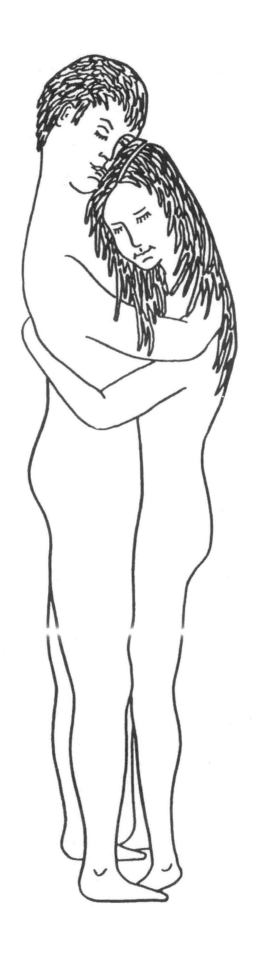

The little sac (testicle) attached to his father's penis contained the seeds (sperm) that would one day join (fertilize) the eggs inside his mother.

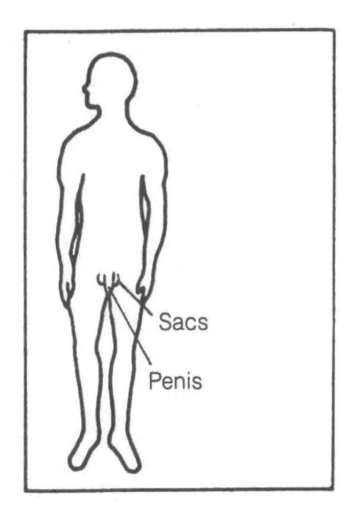

MALE ORGANS (Side View)

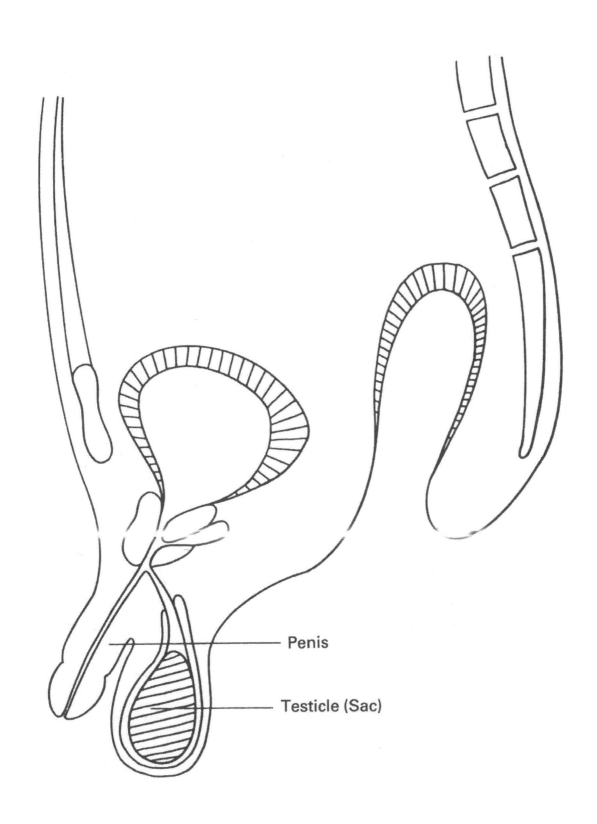

Penis

Testicle (Sac)

Although there were many seeds and many eggs, it took only one seed to enter one egg to begin growth.

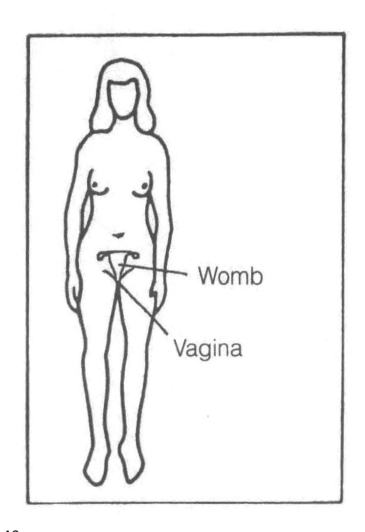

FEMALE ORGANS (Side View)

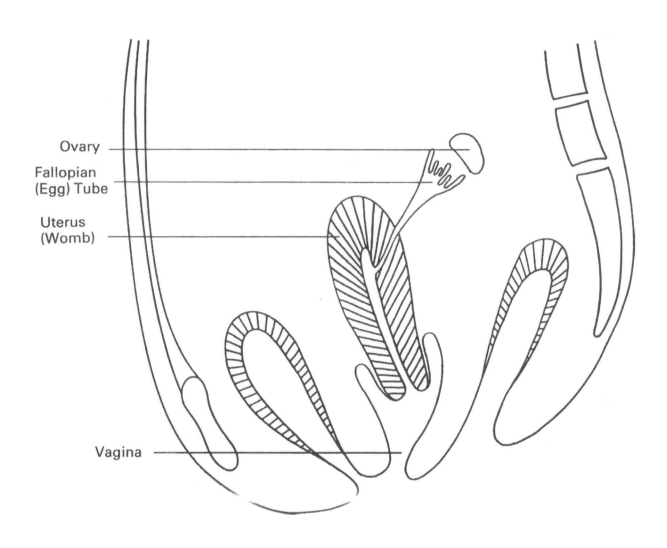

Ovary

Fallopian
(Egg) Tube

Uterus
(Womb)

Vagina

The time was right. His mother's egg was on schedule.

OVARY (Inside)

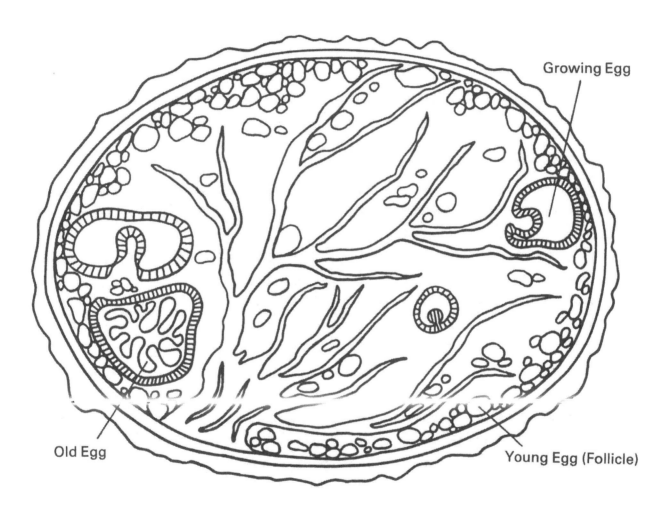

Growing Egg

Old Egg

Young Egg (Follicle)

His father's penis was placed inside his mother's birth canal (vagina).

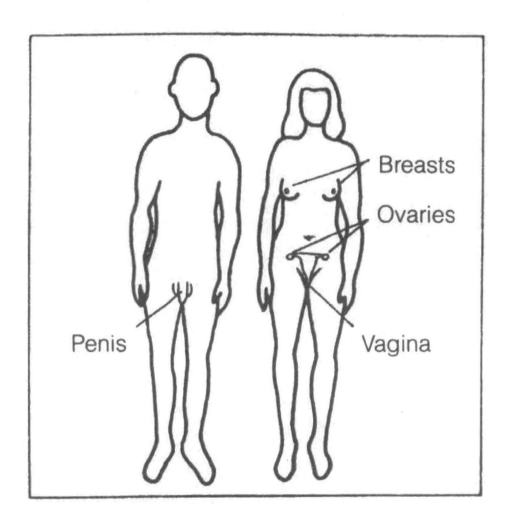

MALE AND FEMALE ORGANS OF REPRODUCTION

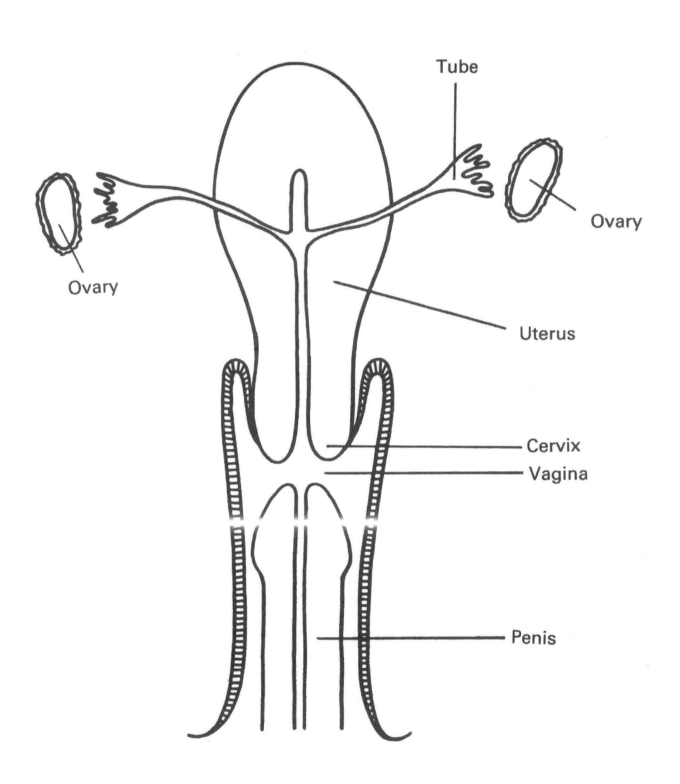

Tube

Ovary

Ovary

Uterus

Cervix

Vagina

Penis

Many seeds were soon released from the little sac.

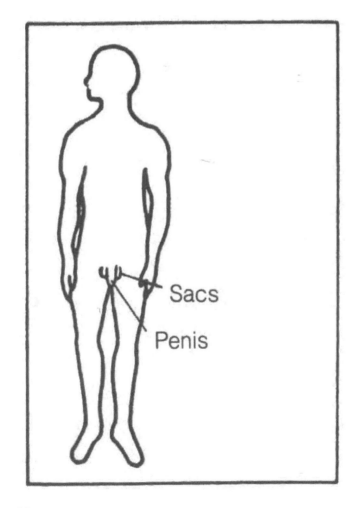

TESTICLE (Inside)

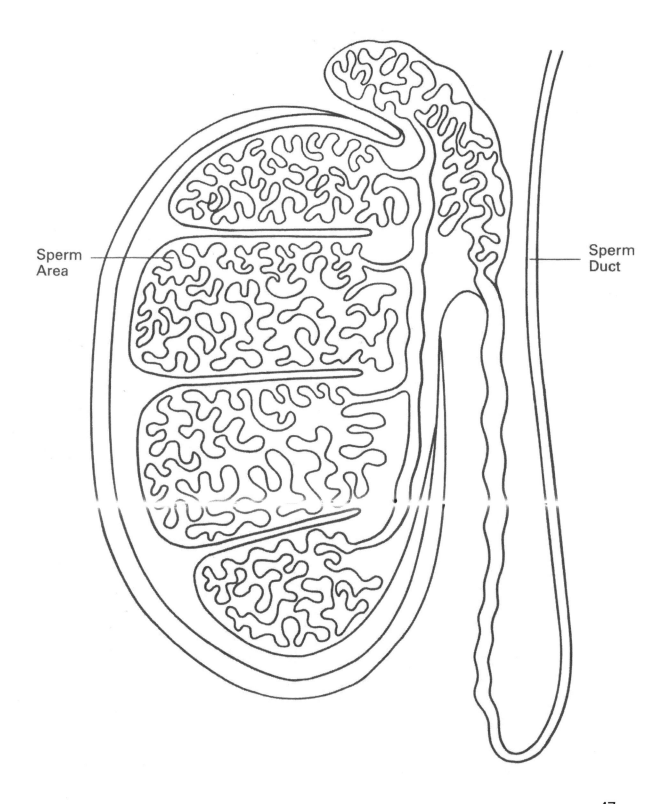

Sperm
Area

Sperm
Duct

One of these seeds, moved along by its tail, made its way through the canal to the mother's egg.

SPERM (MALE SEEDS)

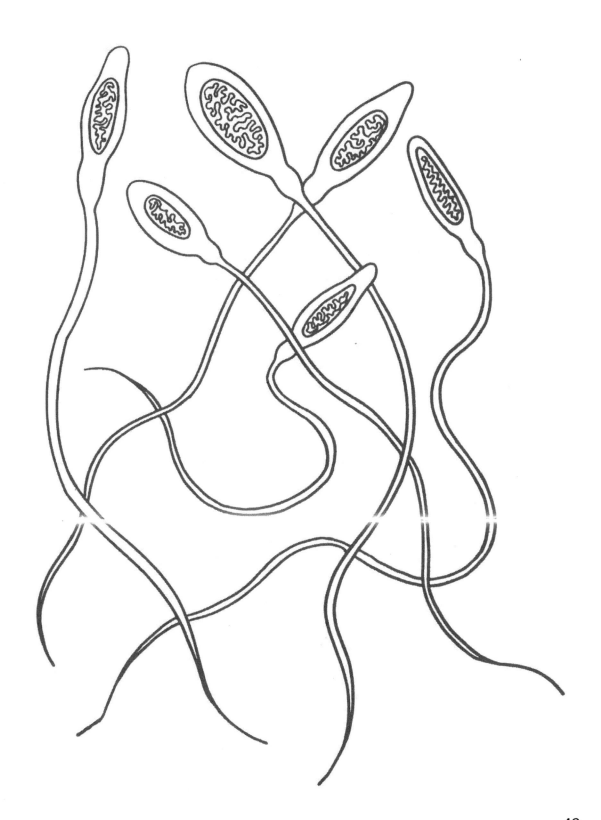

As the seed entered the egg, it lost its tail. Now fertilized, the egg travelled down a tube with an unusual name: the Fallopian Tube. Anton's journey had begun. His mother was pregnant.

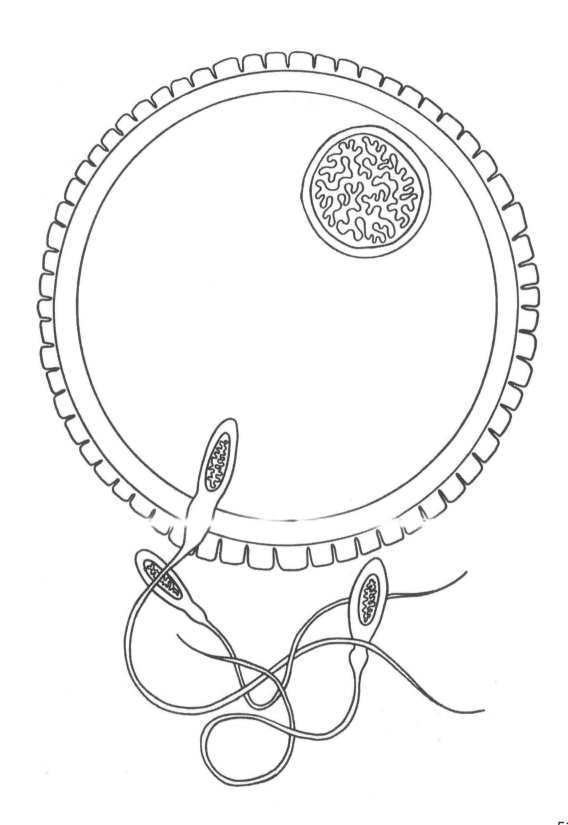

The fertilized egg settled on the wall of the uterus which Anton later heard called the womb...It was a place for him alone ...a wonderful place to grow. It was below and behind his mother's stomach. This would be his cosy, protected resting place while he was prepared for birth in nine months.

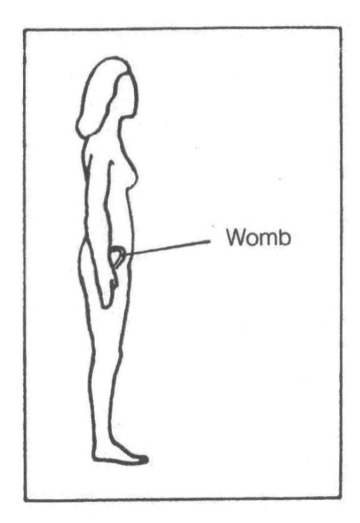

Womb

EARLY SETTING OF FERTILIZED EGG

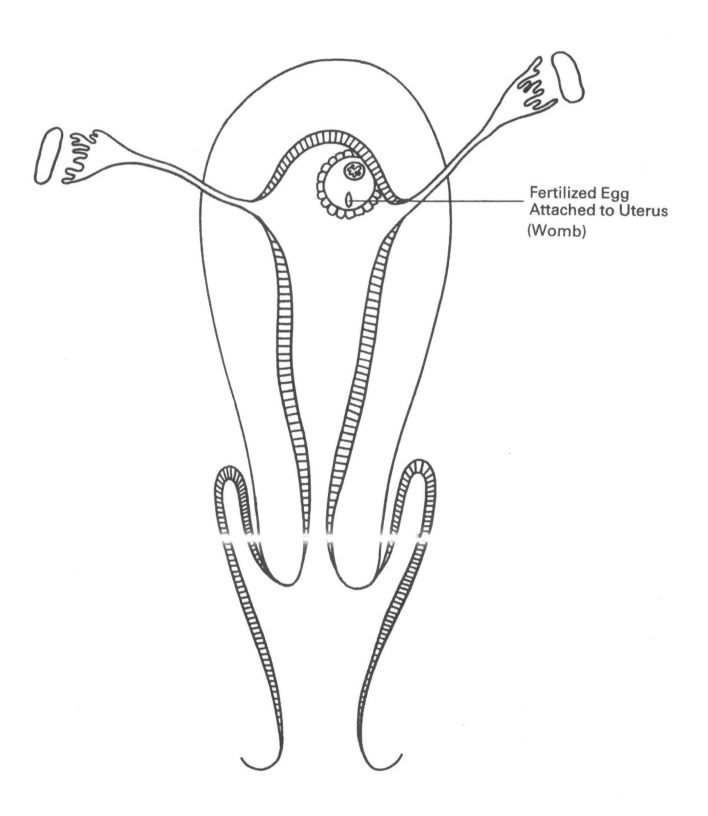

Fertilized Egg
Attached to Uterus
(Womb)

The egg was fed well. It began to divide ... to grow.

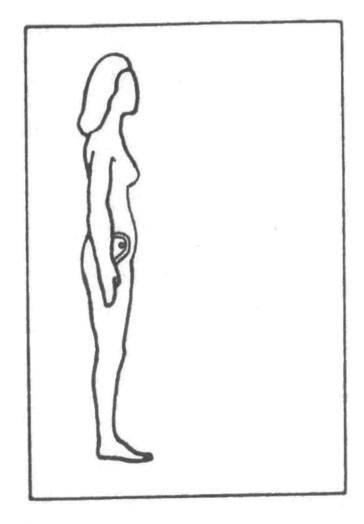

EARLY GROWTH OF FERTILIZED EGG

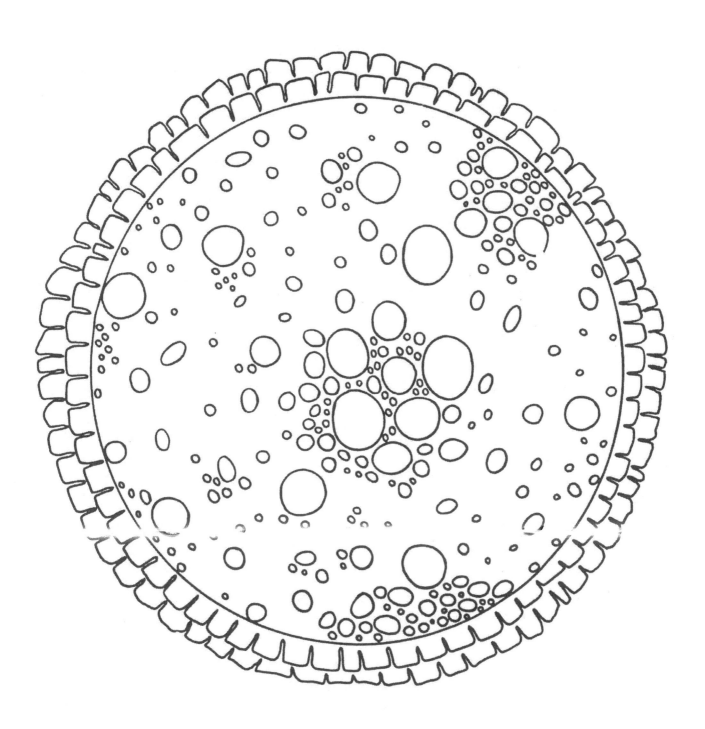

The right food and fresh air, as well as the right thoughts and feelings, were fed to him through a miraculous attachment to the wall of the womb. He had heard them call this attachment the..Placenta...

Anton rested well as he waited his entry into the new world. It was clear that his mother and father wanted him.

He grew, and grew, and grew ...the arms ...legs ... heart ... lungs ... Before he realized it, three months of his nine-month journey had already passed.

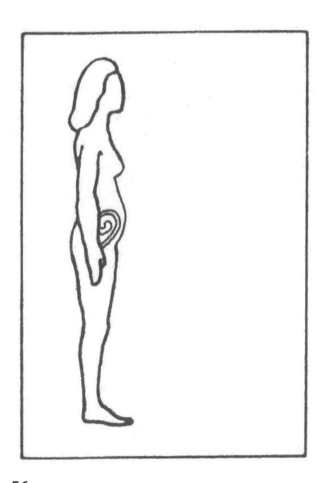

PREGNANCY THREE MONTHS OLD

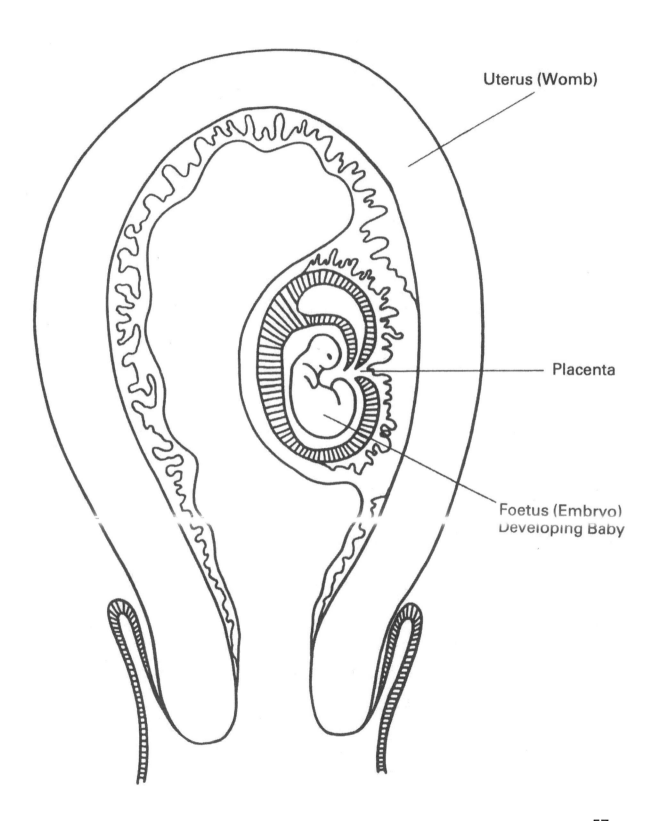

Uterus (Womb)

Placenta

Foetus (Embryo)
Developing Baby

He was now well formed and still growing ... but a bit anxious to get out. Every now and then he'd get enough strength to give a little kick which could be felt outside on his mother's growing tummy (abdomen). This made his mother and father very happy. They were as anxious to meet Anton as Anton was to meet them.

His mother avoided accidents and anything that could bring harm to Anton, for she already loved him very much. As each month passed, he became stronger and stronger, and better and better developed.

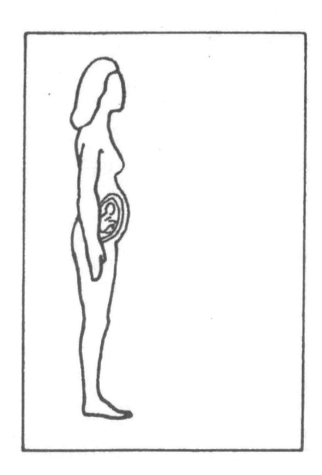

SEVEN MONTH-OLD PREGNANCY

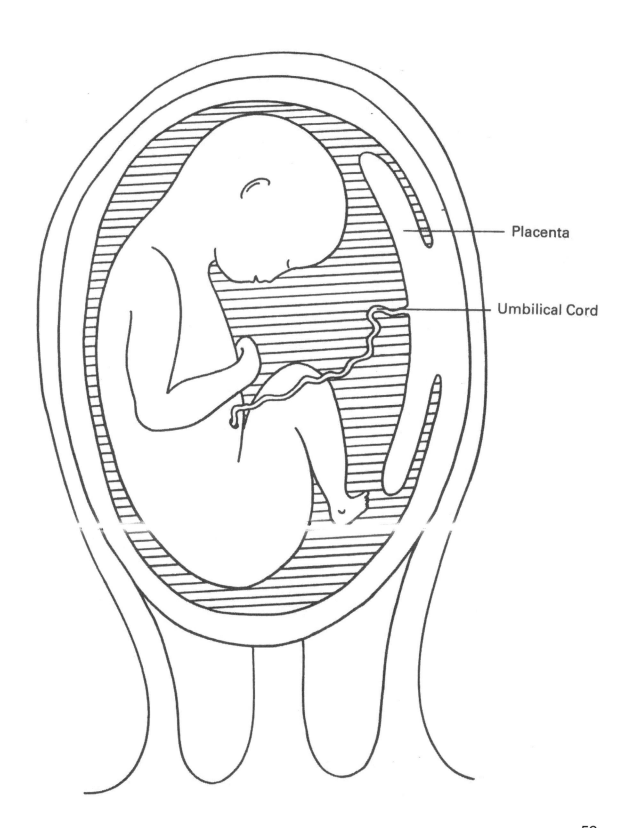

Placenta

Umbilical Cord

He kicked more and more ...and the laughter and love grew between his parents. At last the nine months' waiting was over.

Anton was ready ... ready to be born ... ready to meet his mother and father.

First, his head came out of the womb. The lights were bright. The air was cold.

The rest of his body followed as his mother's birth canal stretched to make room for his exit.

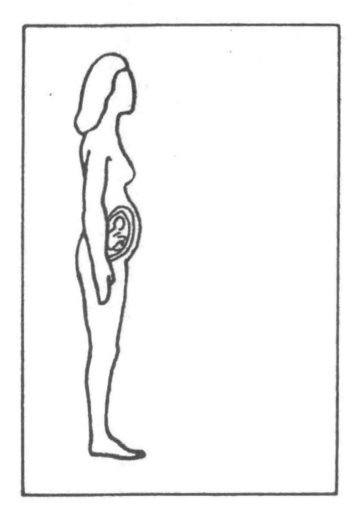

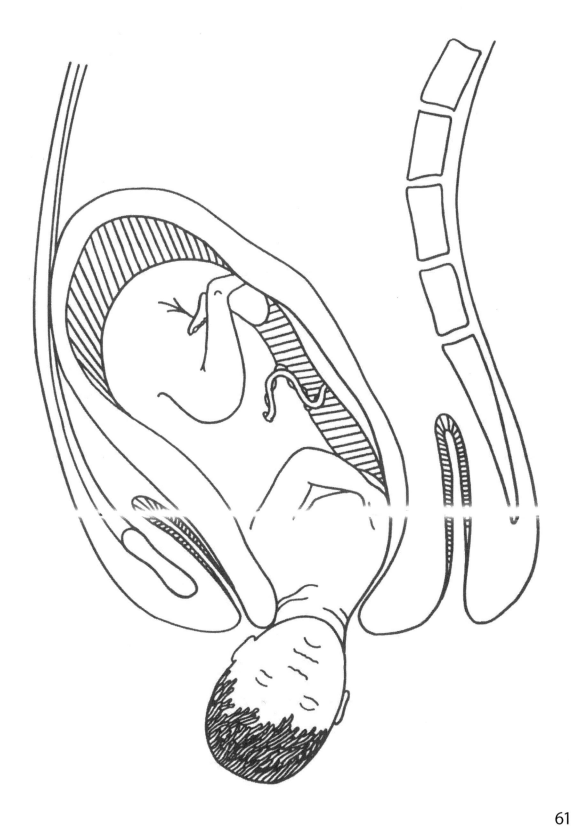

Then came the placenta, attached to a cord which he heard called the "Umbilical Cord". It was tied and cut. It became his belly button.

Anton was born. He was ready for his new adventure. He had everything he needed: health and love of his parents. In his own heart he knew that one day he himself would find that very special kind of love.

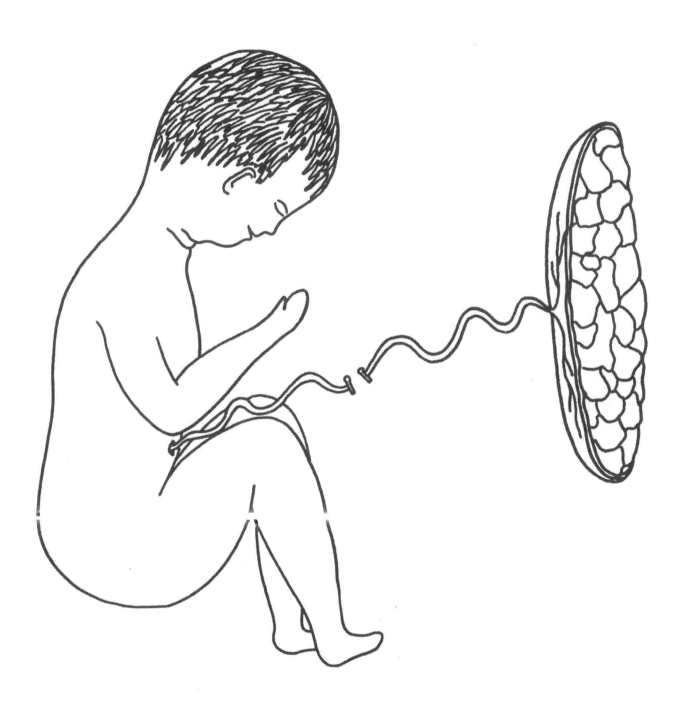

HOW YOUR BODY WORKS

A CHILD'S INTRODUCTION TO THE HUMAN BODY

WONDER
OF LIFE

COLOURING BOOK

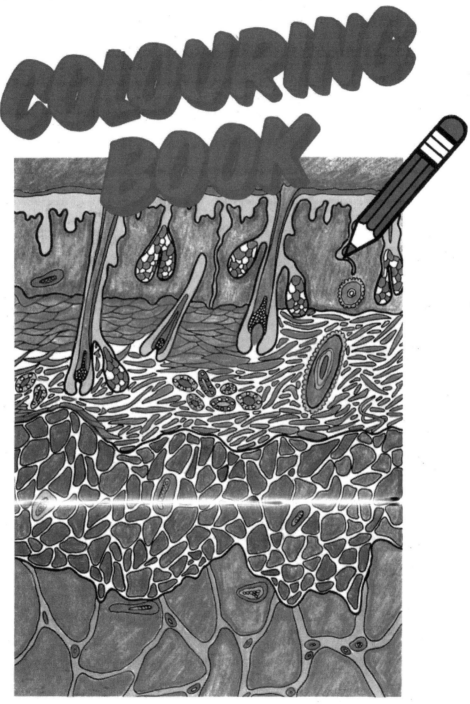

David Sachs M.D.

HOW YOUR BODY WORKS

The purpose of the Wonder of Life series of health educational colouring books about the human body and how it works is to provide children of all ages with the basics of health know ledge and to develop in them the natural sense of self-respect that awaits its rightful colourful expressions.

With these books, children establish awareness of the kaleidoscopic energy in the magnificent patterns and designs that make up their precious human body.

It does not matter what colours the children use: what is important is that they give themselves the conscious attention that healthy bodily parts need to reinforce pride and respect while having a positive healthful effect on the whole body.

Parents and teachers have the responsibility to give children every opportunity to experience daily exposure to each page of this fundamental series.

On every occasion have children actually visualize the exact location, form and function of the specific organ for the day's learning.

While you allow them to freely colour their own expression of this, read aloud the simple text which accompanies each page, emphasizing whatever pleases you at the time.

Through the sharing of this energy between a child and an adult, the maintaining appeal of colouring makes learning about the body meaningful and fun. When this series is used as part of children's everyday activities, you will be rewarded in knowing that they are receiving the foundation for a healthy life, and this will enable every other health habit to be truly effective.

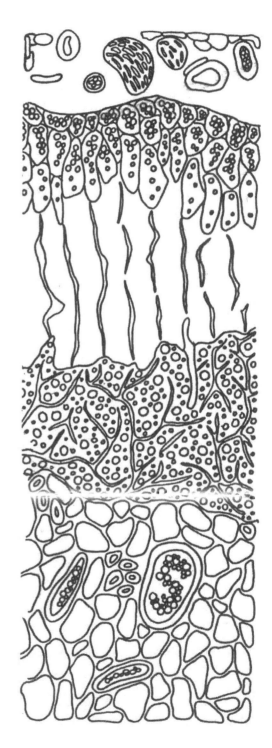

Lining up on the inside curve,
Are special cells that make this nerve.

Through the lens the light reflects,
Forms and colours it detects.

This special sense, a true delight,
needs a pure bloodstream for perfect sight.

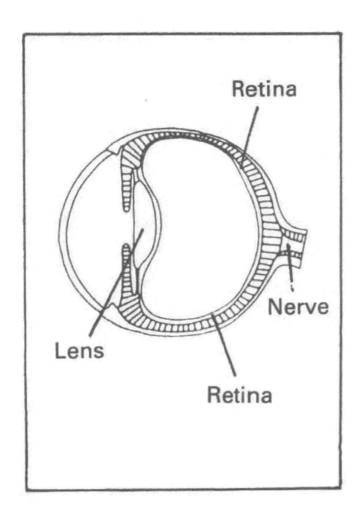

RETINA (BACK OF EYE)

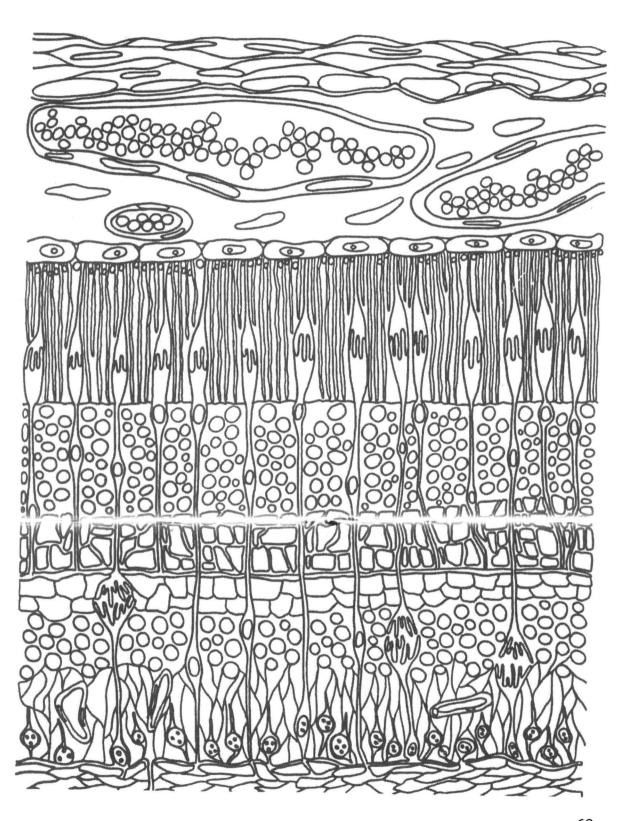

Fluid and cells all reside,
In the tunnels and caves that hide inside.

Sounds of the world are brought within,
From the outer ear where they must begin.

Music and wind made yours to hear,
And sense of balance are gifts of the inner ear.

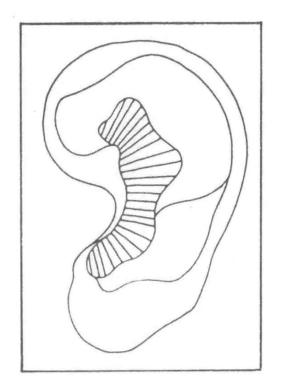
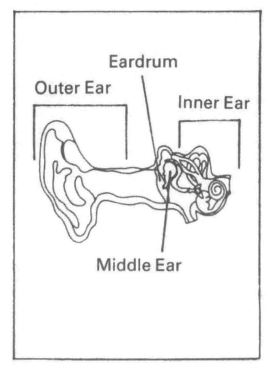

INNER EAR

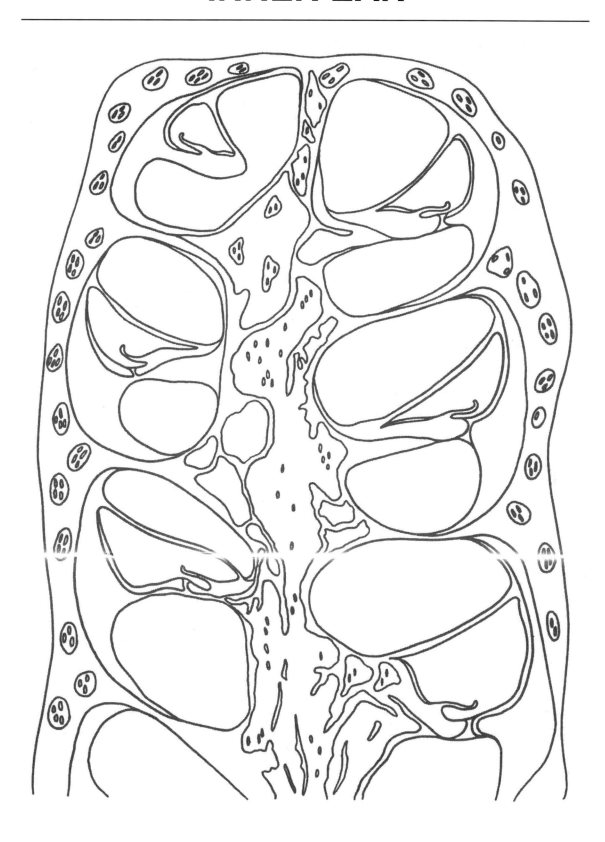

Made of muscle and taste buds many,
It moves about with actions zany.

It helps you swallow, speak and chew,
And hides in your mouth away from view.

Its sense is keen for flavours fine,
You use it almost all the time.

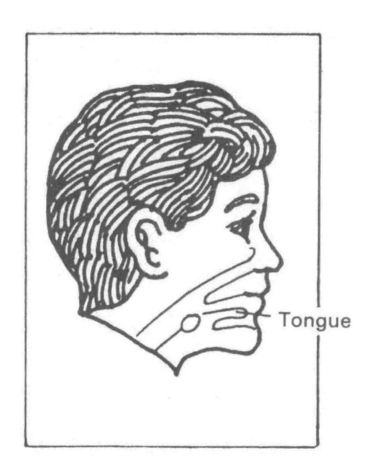

Tongue

TONGUE

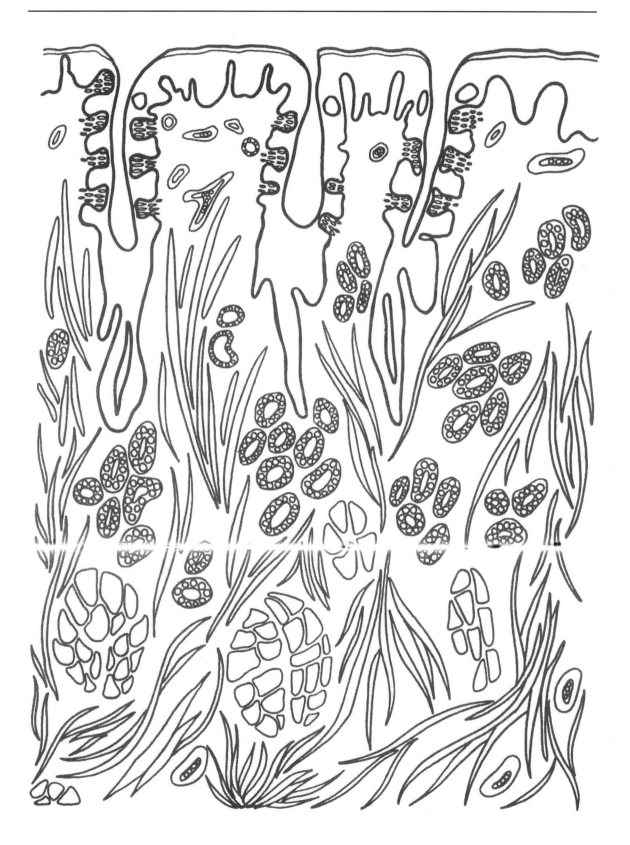

A living computer with will and without,
A centre for thought and feelings no doubt.

Bionic forces control arms, heart and more,
And fill your life with happiness galore.

Thinking by day and dreaming by night,
This magical instrument is yours by right.

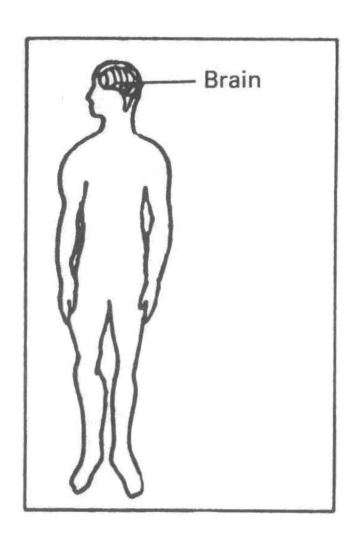

Brain

BRAIN

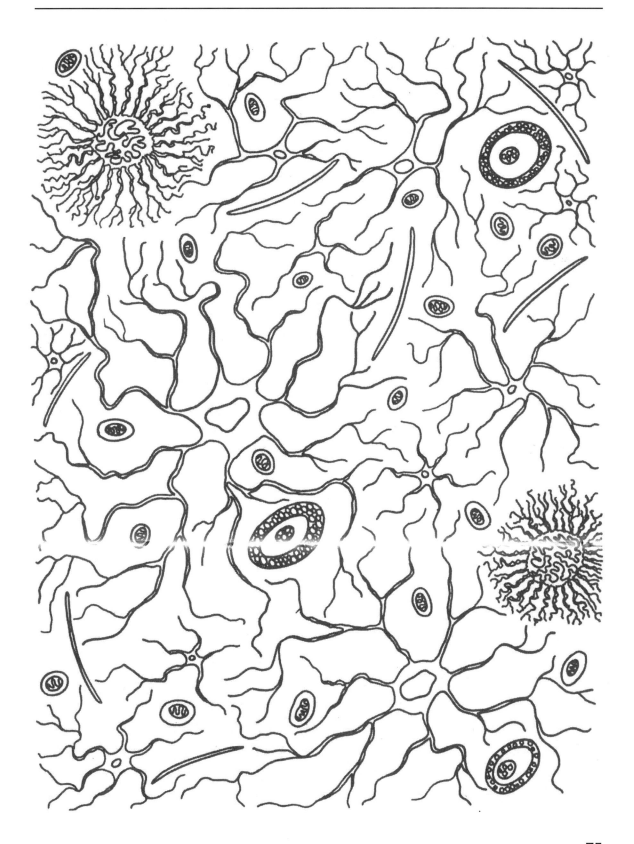

The largest of organs is a busy machine,
It works very hard at keeping you clean.

The blood comes in and the blood goes out,
Some from your heart, but more from about.

Its delicate, intricate cells unite,
To keep you healthy by day and by night.

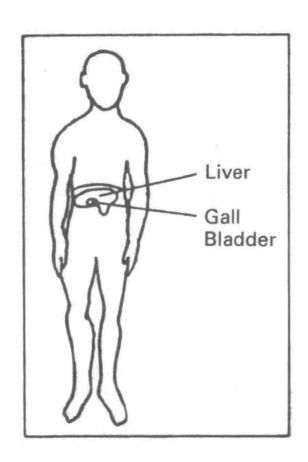

LIVER

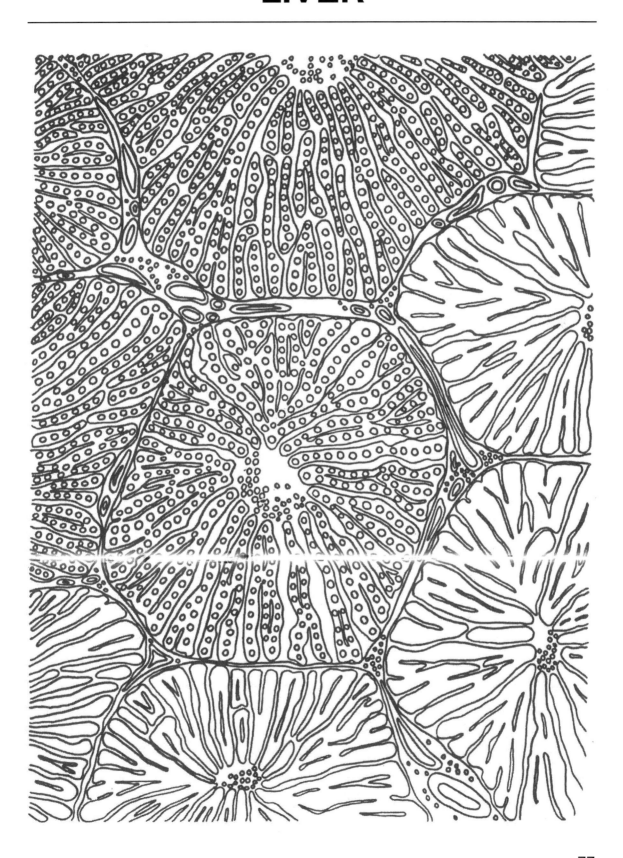

This master gland controller of all,
Sits in a throne ready for call.

From its guarded place beneath the brain,
Messages emerge from your body's gain.

With balance and rhythm it works all day,
To help your body proceed on its way.\

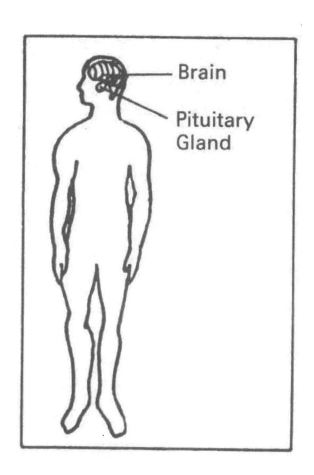

PITUARY GLAND

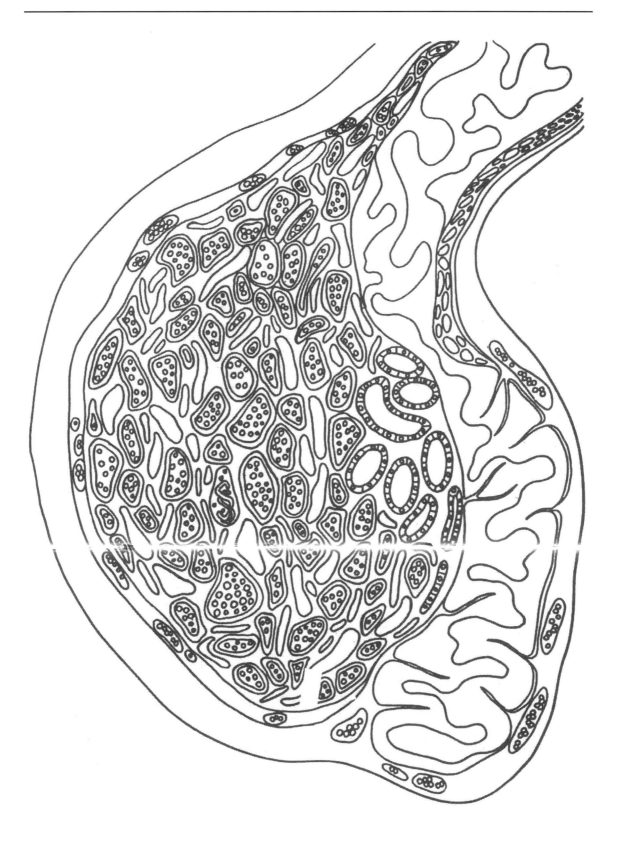

With form and strength challenged by aging,
All the cells are constantly changing
To keep a pace the body insists.
Exercise and diet complete
Make your bones strong, head to feet.

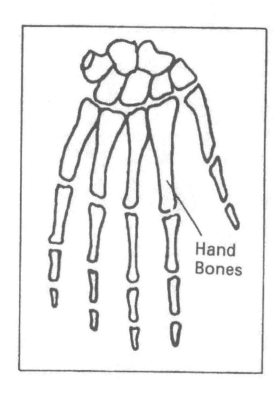

Hand
Bones

BONES

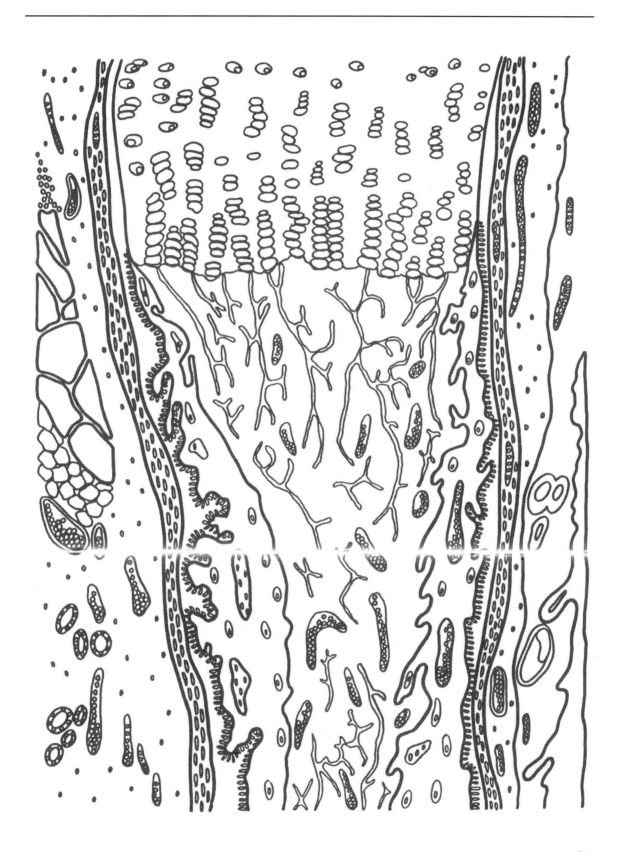

Atop your kidneys two glands rest,
Like three-cornered hats awaiting their test.

They answer all calls, big and small,
To support your stress they give their all.

For this to happen there always must be,
A good supply of Vitamin C.

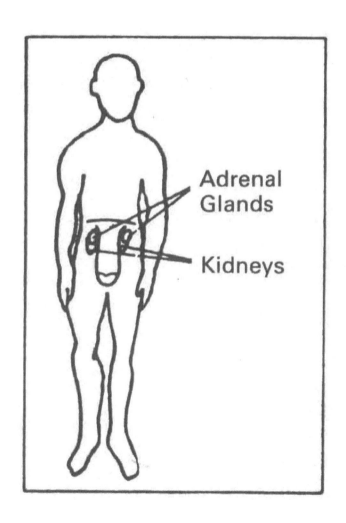

Adrenal Glands

Kidneys

ADRENAL GLANDS

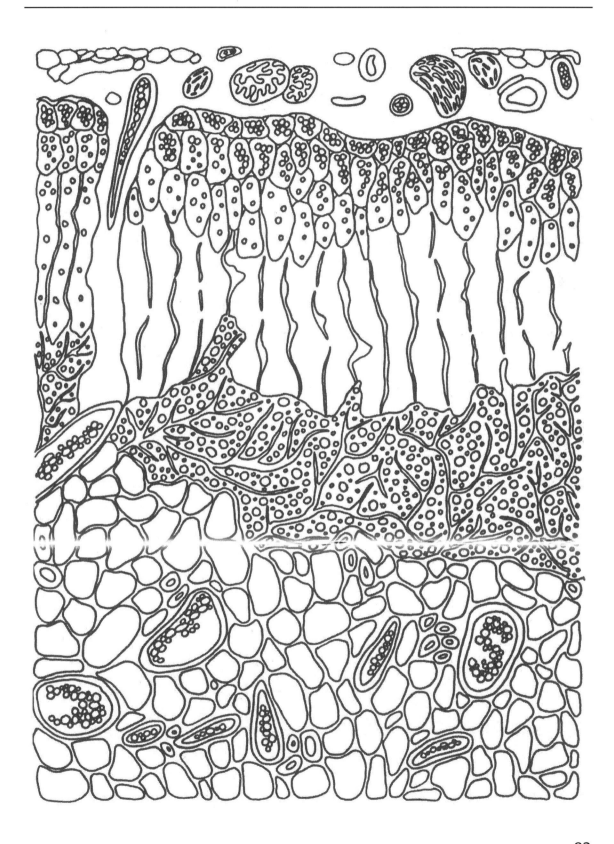

Hard-working organs that never can rest,
The balance of water is part of their test.

In their tireless efforts they remain unshaken,
And anything harmful from the body is taken.

From your blood they will filter the things you don't need,
And of the salt in your body they also take heed.

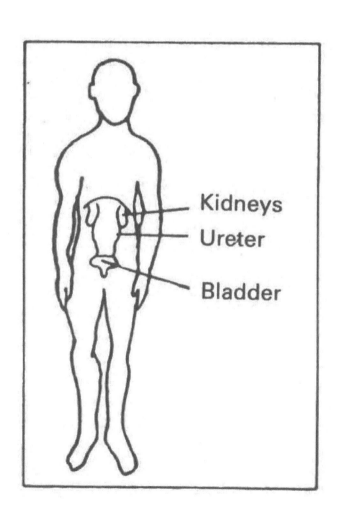

KIDNEYS

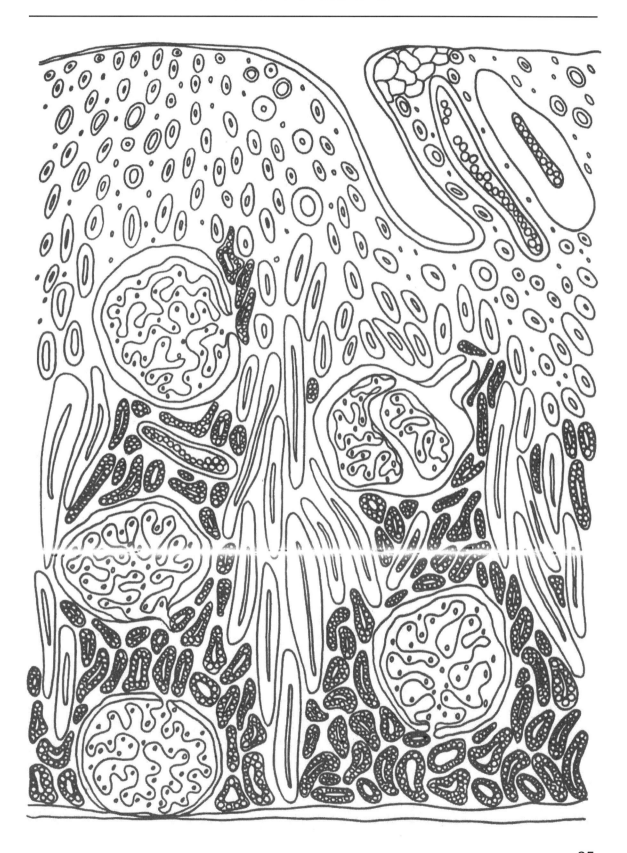

Inside the centres of your bones there dwells,
The marrow that works to supply the cells.
The red blood cells have a critical quest,
For carrying oxygen is what they do best.
To fight infection is the white cells' care,
While platelets for clotting the blood are there.

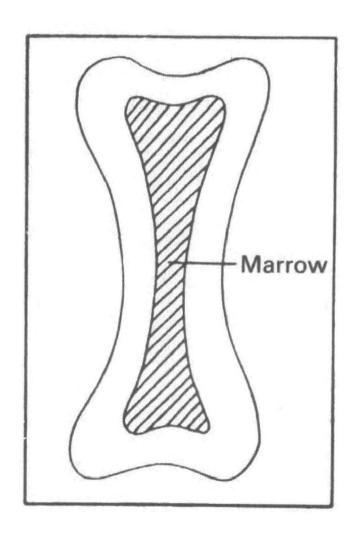

BLOOD CELLS

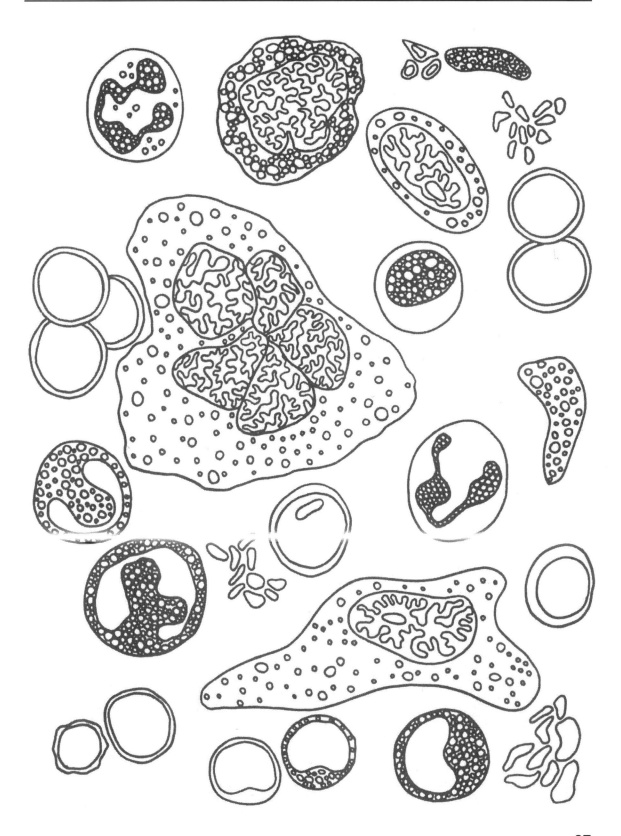

This gland rests in the upper chest,
Awaiting a chance to do its best.

Large at birth, then shrinking in size,
That it has secrets no one denies.

There are many tasks that may be involved,
Immunity is one which has not yet been solved.

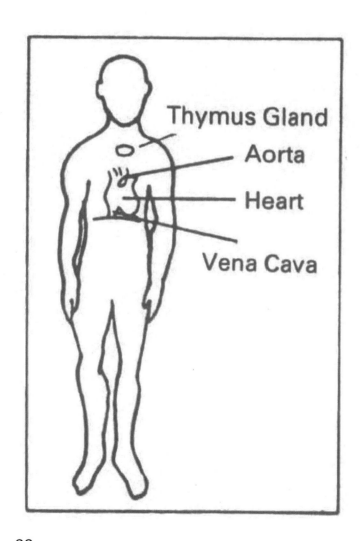

Thymus Gland

Aorta

Heart

Vena Cava

THYMUS GLAND

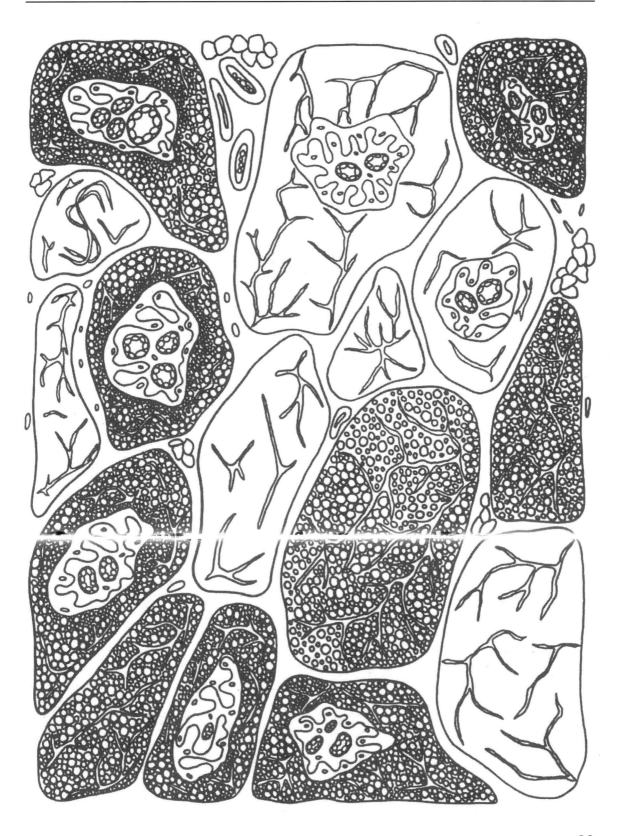

When food, juice, or water you swallow,
This sac, big or small, is no longer hollow.

It gets things you eat ready to go
For a journey beyond to the intestine below.

With acids strong and enzymes right,
It can rumble and ache, so don't be uptight.

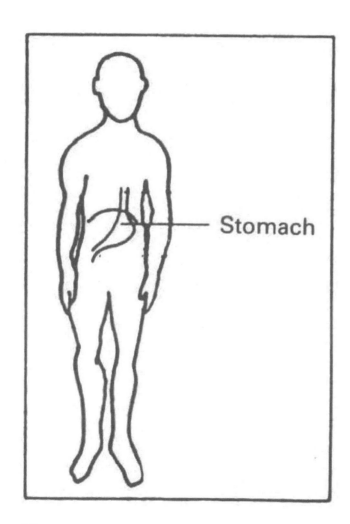

Stomach

STOMACH

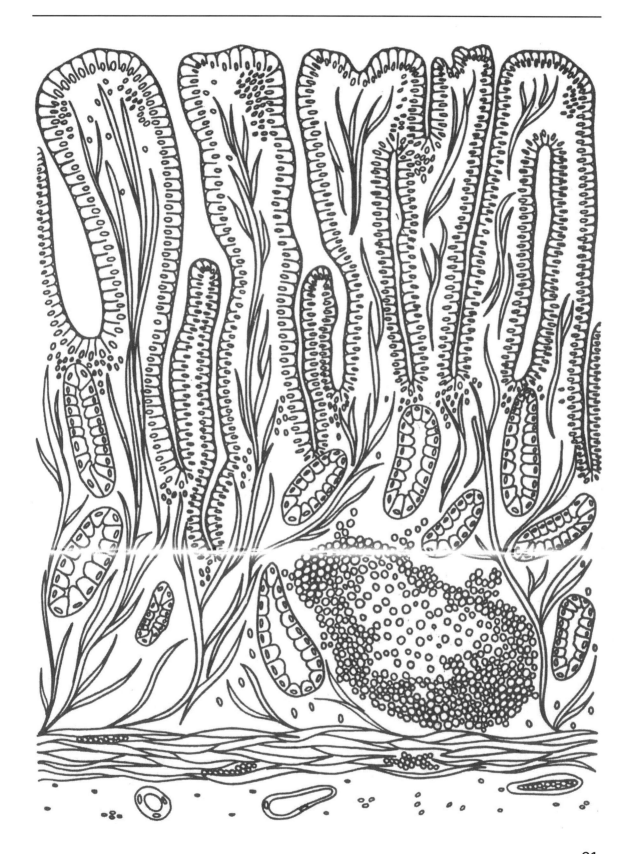

Back in your throat, on the left and the right,
Two glands lie in waiting, infection to fight.

These pillars guard as protective screens,
To make air, food and water clean.

From birth until twelve they continue to grow,
They were once thought a pest but now we all know.

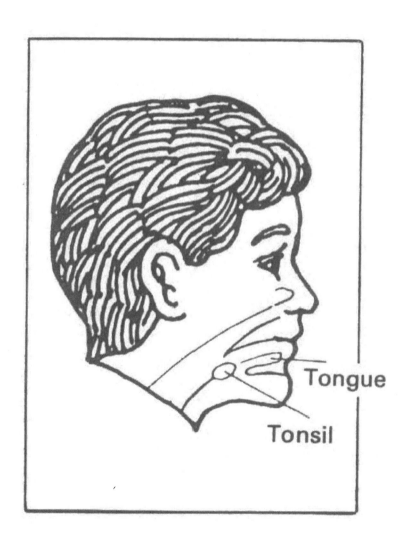

Tongue

Tonsil

TONSILS

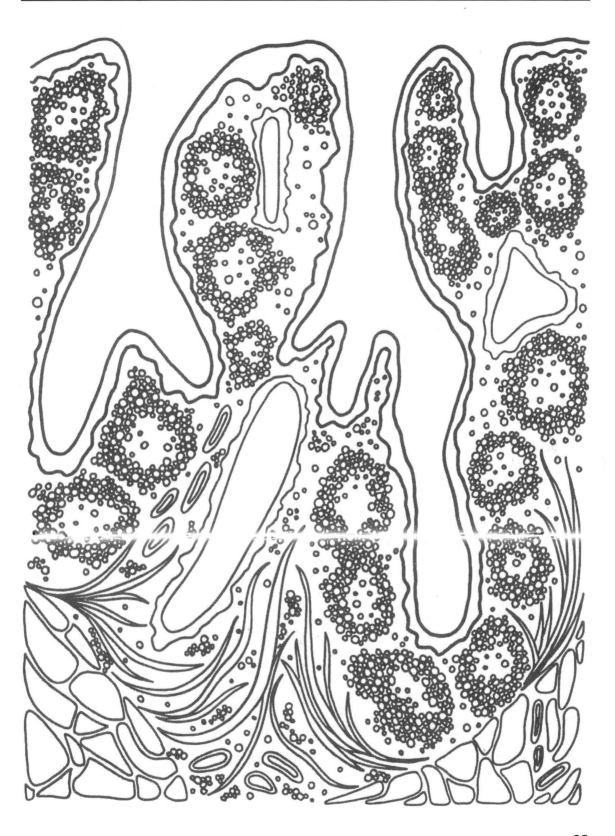

Beneath the jaw, inside the cheek,
Three pairs of glands deal with all that you eat.

Into the mouth their juices come,
To protect your teeth, and moisten the gums.

Amounts large or small automatically flow,
Just why this occurs the glands seem to know.

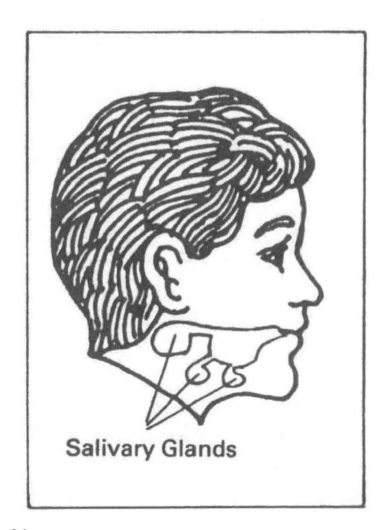

Salivary Glands

SALIVARY GLANDS

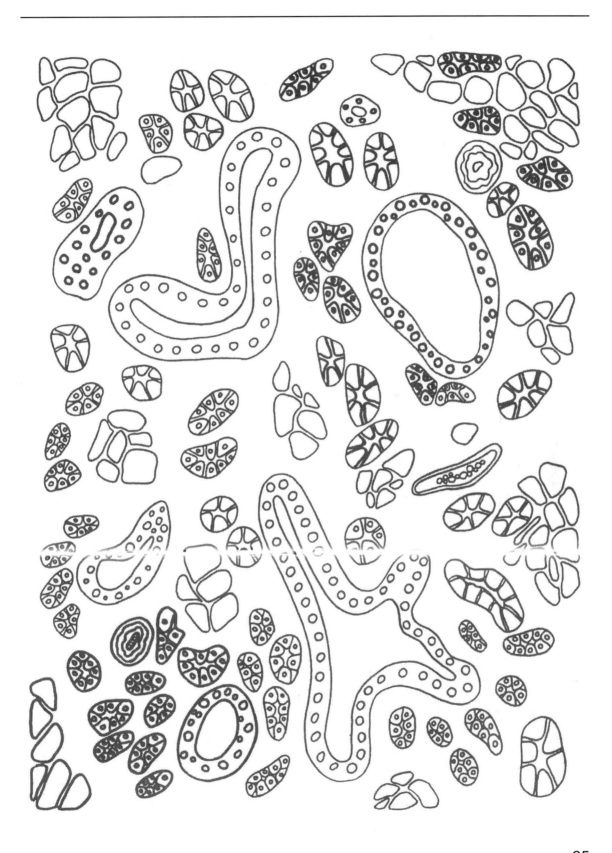

An envelope thick and thin about,
The skin protects from what is without.

It has hairs and glands of oil and sweat,
And nerves to tell warm, sharp and wet.

In all its colours- yellow, black, red and white
It is at its best with careful sunlight.

SKIN

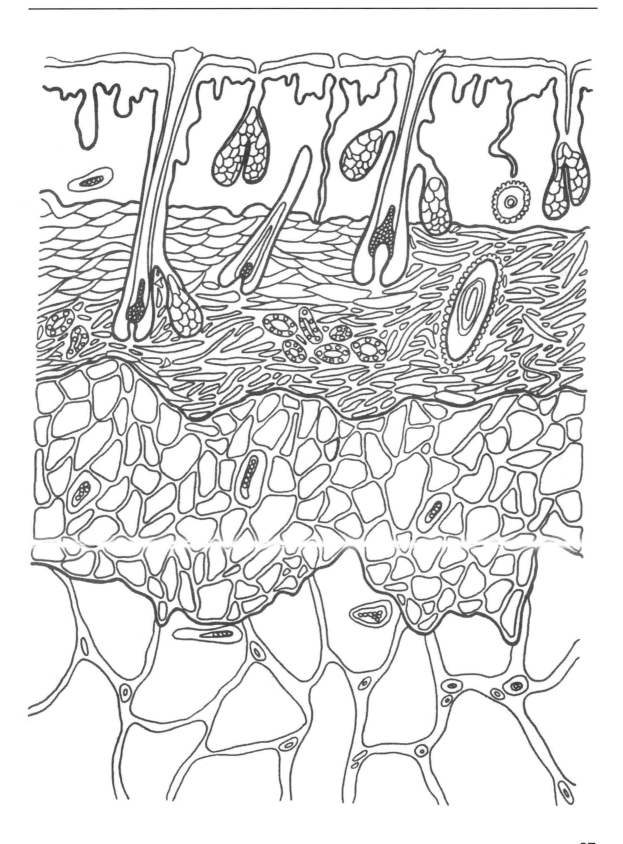

HOW YOUR GENES WORK
A CHILD'S INTRODUCTION TO THE HUMAN BODY

WONDER OF LIFE

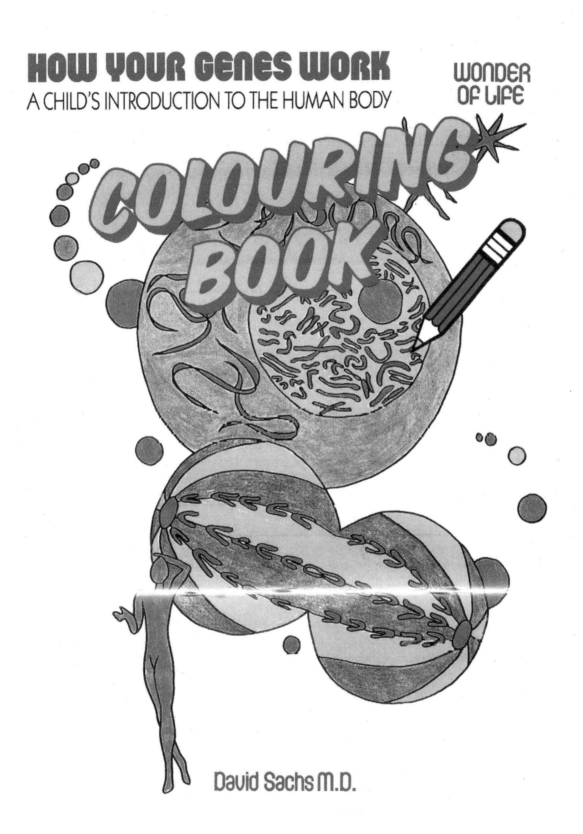

COLOURING BOOK

David Sachs M.D.

HOW YOUR GENES WORK

The purpose of the Wonder of Life series of health education colouring books about the human body and how it works, is to provide children of all ages with the basics of health knowledge and to develop in them the natural sense of self-respect that awaits its rightful colourful expressions.

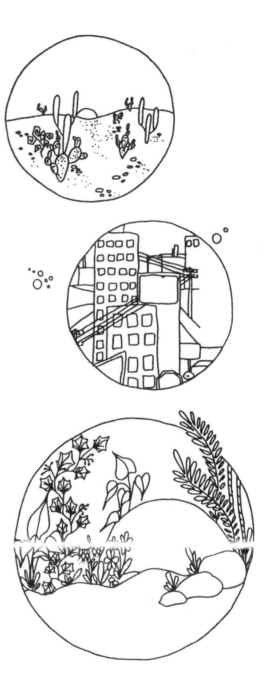

With these books, children establish awareness of the kaleidoscopic energy in the magnificent patterns and designs that make up their precious human body.

It does not matter what colours the children use: what is important is that they give themselves the conscious attention that healthy bodily parts need to reinforce pride and respect while having a positive healthful effect on the whole body.

Parents and teachers have the responsibility to give children every opportunity to experience daily exposure to each page of this fundamental series.

On every occasion have children actually visualize the exact location, form and function of the specific organ for the day's learning.

While you allow them to freely colour their own expression of this, read aloud the simple text which accompanies each page, emphasizing whatever pleases you at the time.

Through the sharing of this energy between a child and an adult, the entertaining appeal of colouring makes learning about the human body meaningful and fun.

When this series is used as part of children's everyday activities, you will be rewarded in knowing that they are receiving the foundation for a healthy life, and this will enable every other health habit to be truly effective.

I am …You are …
a story of how you came to be You …
a human mosaic …
a living symphony. •

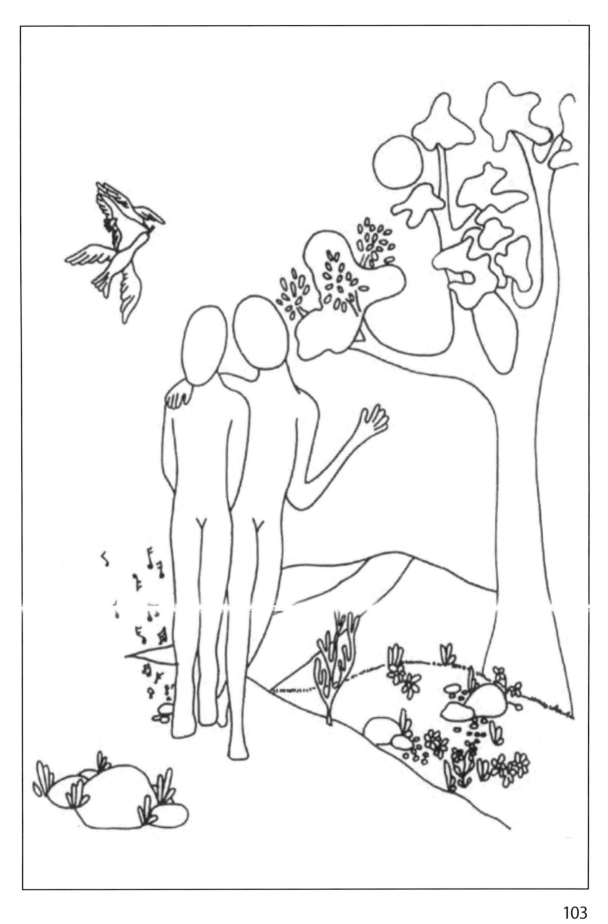

Every cell in your body contains a programme ...
a set of instructions (known as DNA)
with endless combinations
that guarantee you will be you ...
a unique person.

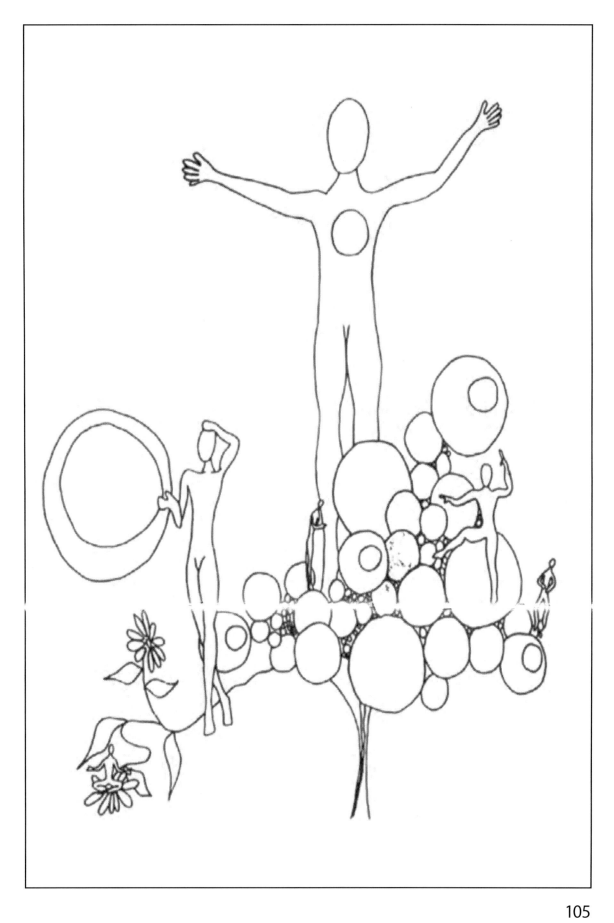

You are a song ...
with melodies and rhythms
written in your genes ... genes inherited
half from your father,
half from your mother ...
also, from their parents and their parents
and their parents ... all the way back.

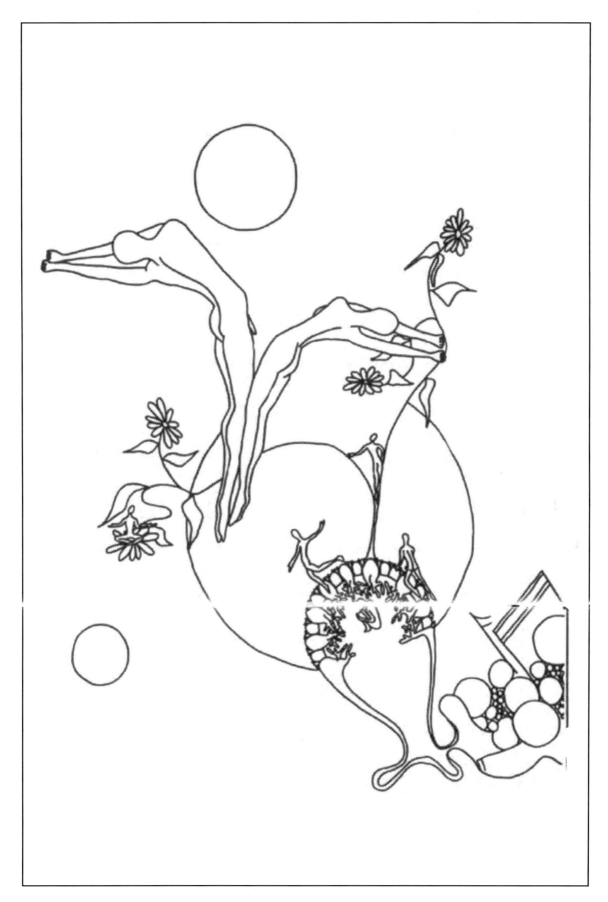

107

You are an orchestra
with 46 musicians (genes) working together
to produce a life influenced by
your space and your time,
days and generations, births and rebirths ...
and the concern and love
of your entire family tree.

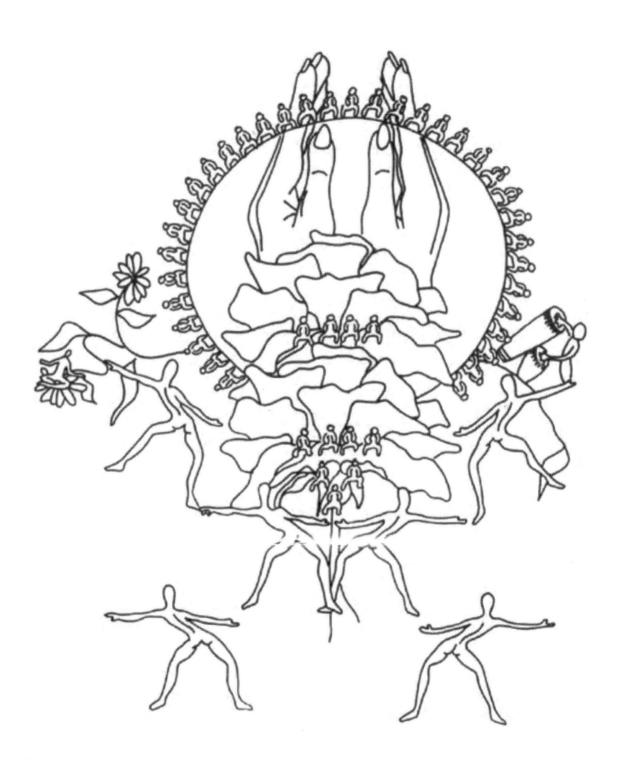

You are composed, like music,
of both strong and weak elements
that in the tiny miracle world of genes ...
in chromosomes ...in cells ...
in you ... create melodies
of human life and being AND

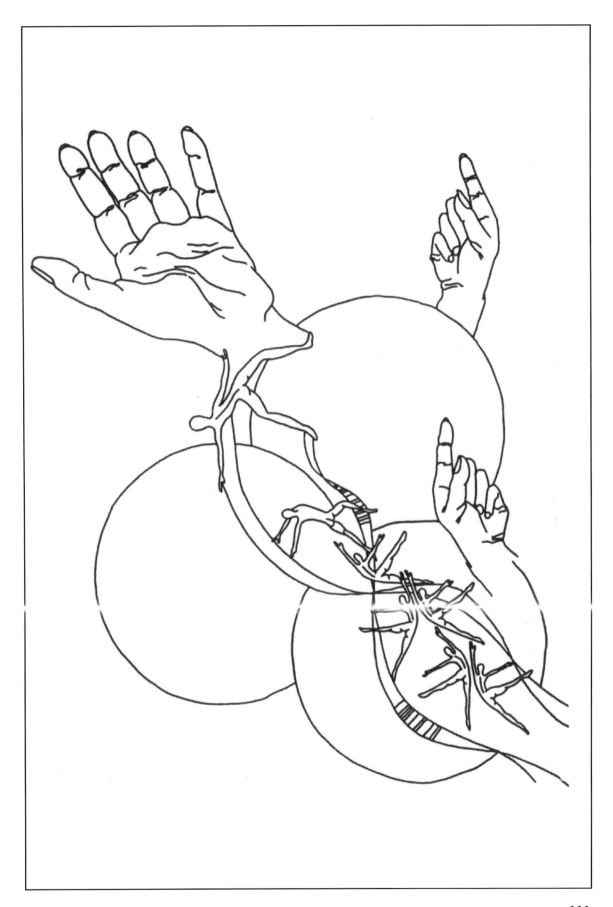

compare, mix and contrast
the best combinations present
in your parents' special mixture.
Sets of genes, like stereo speakers,
come in pairs (one from each parent)
and, when possible, the strongest associations,
like the clearest harmonies, are produced.

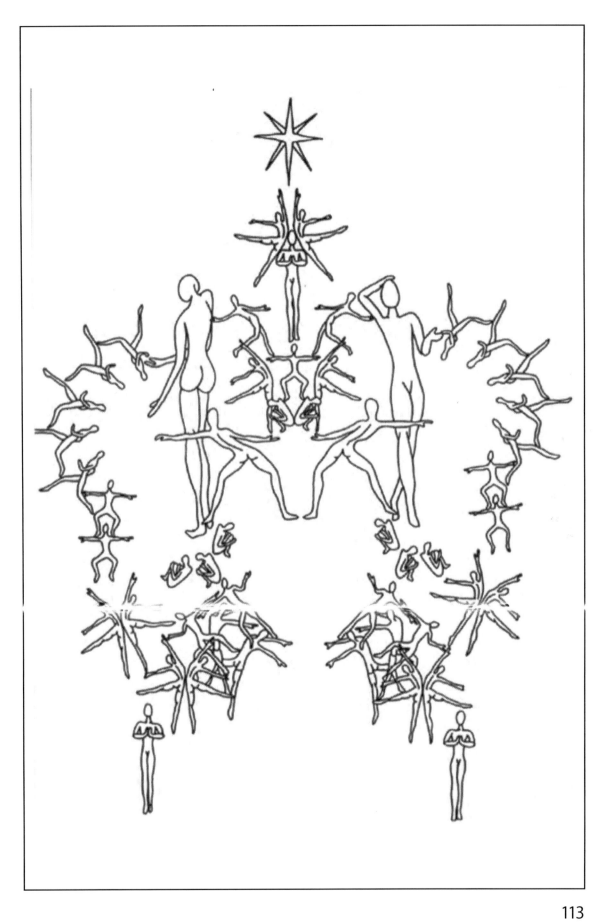

Physical, mental, and emotional characteristics are passed from one generation to the next.

Atuning your inheritance by acquiring the all-important knowledge of the human body,you can become the conductor for your own unique harmony through your wonderful orchestra.

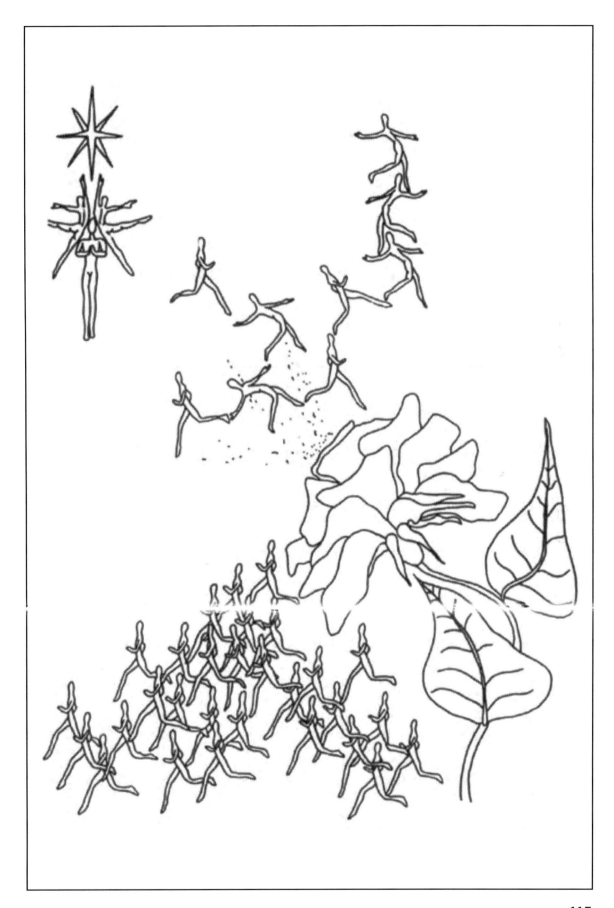

All life, plant and animal alike,
has fantastic variations ...
genetic possibilities ...
it is likely for a boy to resemble his mother ...
a girl to resemble her father.

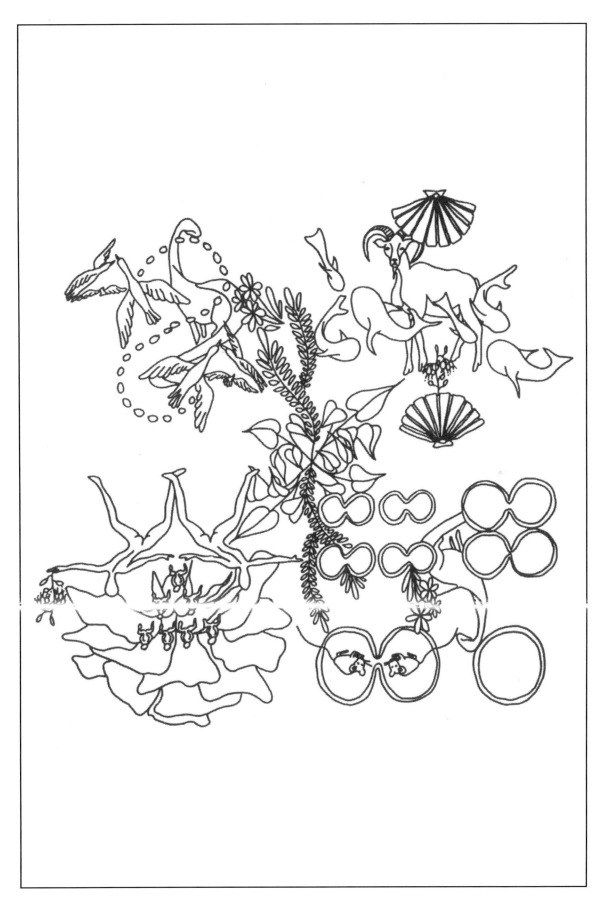

The unknown structures
of our genes and chromosomes
that provide the score for our symphony,
that define our inheritance,
are just now being discovered.

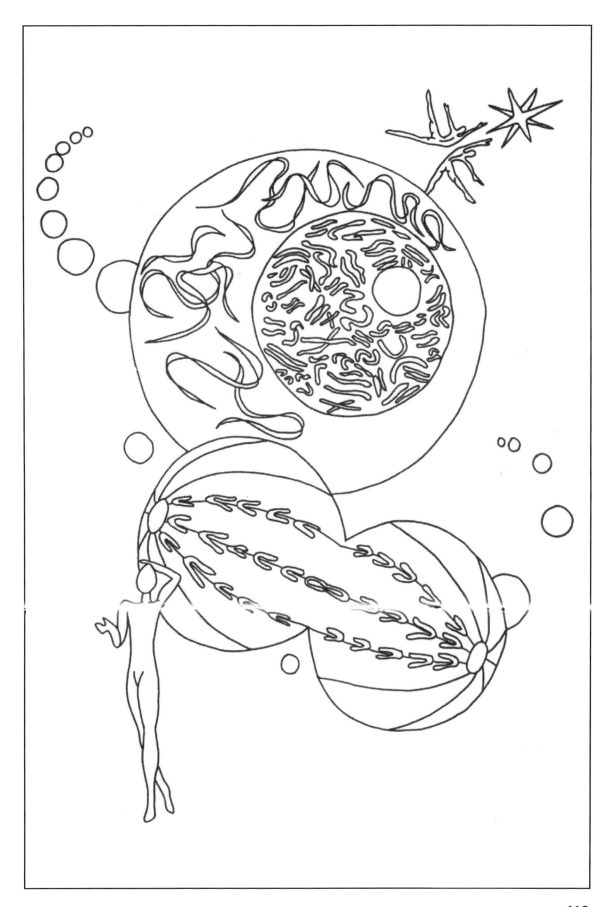

As there are thousands of melodies
so there is unlimited potential,
with great differences between every person ...
even brothers and sisters
can be as different as total strangers.

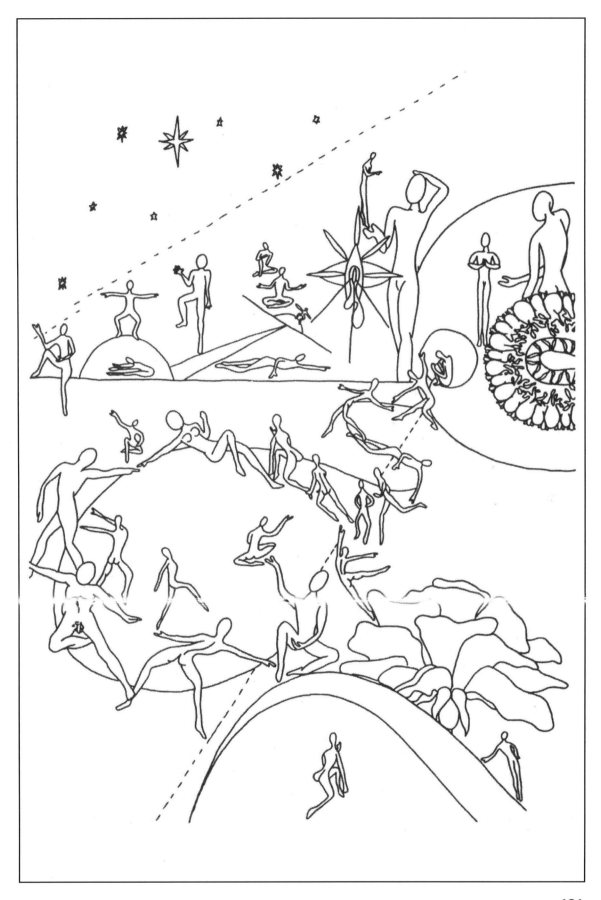

Like seating an orchestra,
the violins here, the drums there ...
each piece in its place ...
elements you inherit and wish to share ...
hair colour ... skin colour ...
can be imagined.

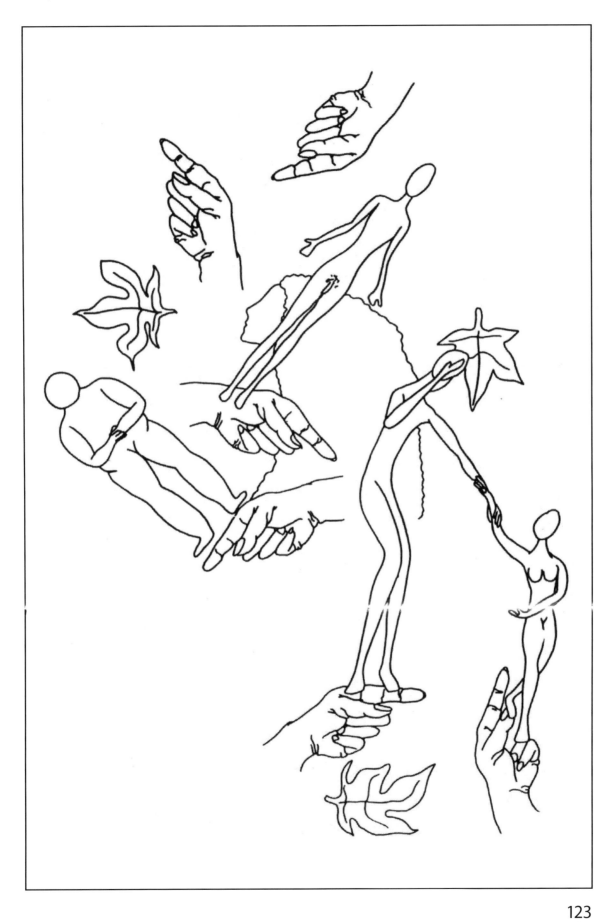

Your 46 musicians are playing together
for the first time,
and only the conductor knows how
they will sound.
Others' expectations of you might
not really be you.

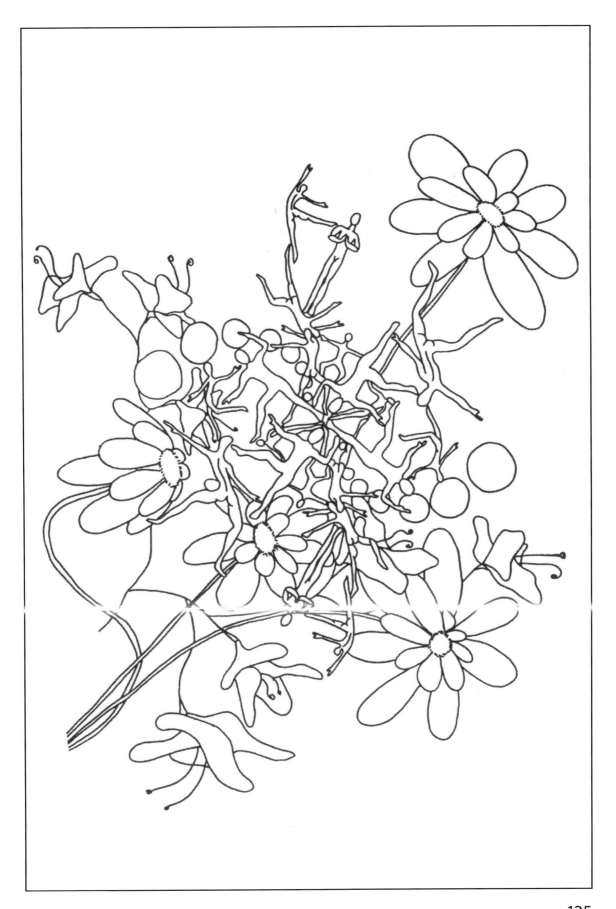

125

**Where you and your ancestors
have lived and for how long ...
the environment, past and present ...
affects your characteristics throughout your life
and in future generations.**

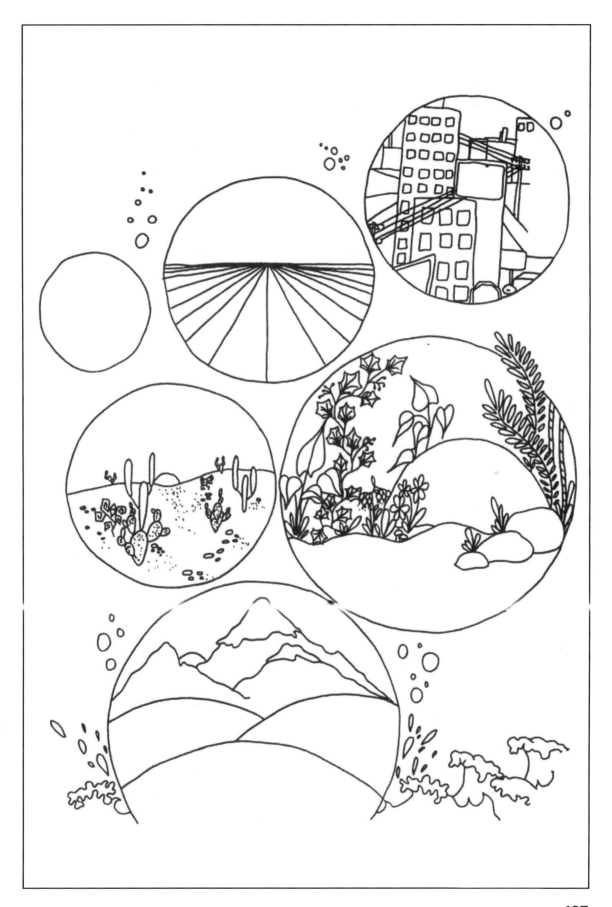

127

Like a finely tuned, living instrument ...
your response to the flow of changes
in your "world/environment/habitat"...
your adaptability to the constant movement
of "living/growing/being" ...
keeps you in harmony with your own genetic
timing and direction.

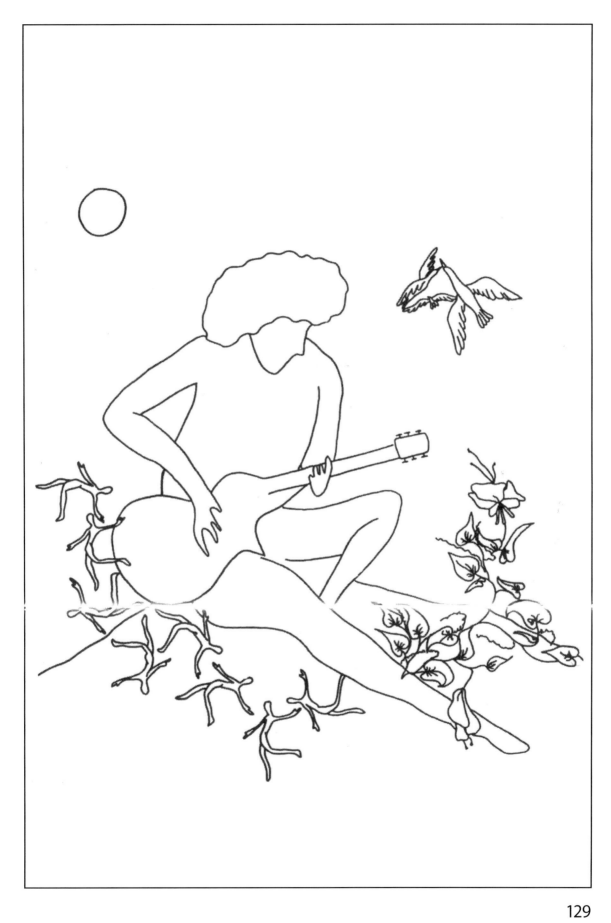

Selectivity and choice
Adaptability like a voice ...
Calling you to listen to your genes.

Heredity and concern
Possibilities done to a turn ...
This is what genetics really means.

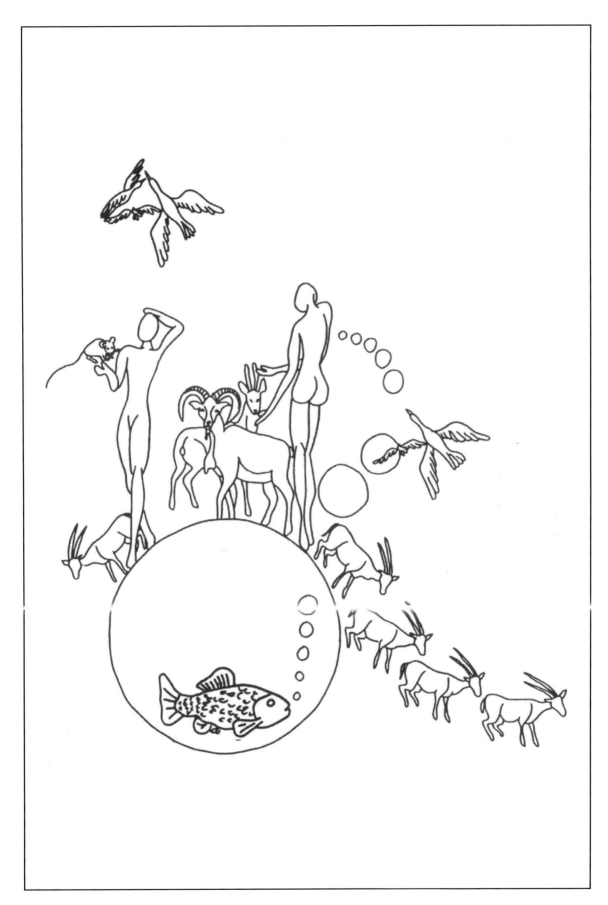

Printed in the United States
By Bookmasters